Kaori Haishi is an essayist and saké journalist, and chairwoman of the Japan Saké Association. She was born in Nerima in Tokyo in 1966, and graduated from the Department of German Language and Literature, Nihon University College of Humanities and Sciences. She then worked as a radio reporter and a journalist for a weekly women's magazine. She visits saké breweries and shōchū and Awamori makers all over Japan to write articles for various media. She also gives talks, seminars, and recipe suggestions for pairing saké and food. She set up the Japan Saké Association in 2015, training saké experts to international standards, and running saké events at various locations in Japan.

Dr Shinichi Asabe is a former associate professor at the Department of Gastroenterology, Internal Medicine, Jichi Medical University Saitama Medical Center. After he graduated from the Faculty of Medicine at the University of Tokyo in 1990, he worked at the University of Tokyo Hospital, and Department of Gastroenterology at Toranomon Hospital. He is mainly involved in viral hepatitis studies at the National Cancer Center Japan, and after work at the Jichi Medical University Hospital, he studied the immunology of hepatitis at the Scripps Research Institute in San Diego, US. Back in Japan in 2010, he started to work at the Department of Gastroenterology, Internal Medicine, Jichi Medical University Saitama Medical Center. Currently he is based at AbbVie GK. He specialises in hepatology and virology, and loves wine, saké and beer.

The Japanese Guide to Healthy Drinking

Advice from a Sake-loving Doctor on
How Alcohol Can Be Good for You

**Kaori Haishi and
Dr Shinichi Asabe**

ROBINSON

ROBINSON

SAKEZUKI ISHI GA OSHIERU SAIKO NO NOMIKATA
Copyright © 2017 Kaori Haishi, Shinichi Asabe
English translation rights arranged with Nikkei Business Publications, Inc.
through Japan UNI Agency, Inc., Tokyo.

First published in Great Britain in 2021 by Robinson

Translated by Motoko Tamamuro and Jonathan Clements

1 3 5 7 9 8 6 4 2

The moral right of the author has been asserted.

A CIP catalogue record for this book
is available from the British Library

ISBN: 978-1-47214-456-0

Typeset in Minion Pro by SX Composing DTP, Rayleigh, Essex
Printed and bound in Great Britain by Clays Ltd, Elcograf S.p.A.

Papers used by Robinson are from well-managed forests
and other responsible sources

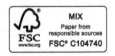

Robinson
An imprint of
Little, Brown Book Group
Carmelite House
50 Victoria Embankment
London EC4Y 0DZ

An Hachette UK Company
www.hachette.co.uk

www.littlebrown.co.uk

Contents

Introduction

'Drink in moderation and live a longer life.'

That's what people say, and probably for the same reason, which is that many habitual drinkers, myself included, can be over-confident. It doesn't matter so much when you are young, and a medical check-up is unlikely to be something to be afraid of. But as we get older, all sorts of values – our y-GTP, our triglyceride levels, our uric acid count – can start to bother us.

But still, we don't stop drinking. We might get anxious, wondering if it's really okay to keep drinking like we used to, but when the city lights beckon, we hit the town and say: 'Hey, let's go for a pint!'

Alcoholic drinks are tasty and enjoyable. But can we really keep up such a pace of drinking without worrying about our health?

I was nearing fifty, and fretting about such issues whenever I went out drinking, when I was asked to write a book on the subject of 'drinking and health'. To tell the truth, I am not an expert in a medical field, but I do have an in-depth experience of how drinkers actually feel. So I thought I would go to the doctors and the experts with a set of simple questions and concerns common among boozers. This book is the result.

Many a tippler will say that doctors only advise us that we should drink in moderation. And sure, that is true, but most of the doctors and experts I interviewed turned out to like a drink themselves. In other words, they understand us very well. And that prompted them to tell me, with the benefit of their own experiences, how we can lead long and healthy lives without giving up drinking altogether.

In the course of my interviews, one thing became clear – alcohol can harm you or help you, depending on how you drink it.

As I explain in Chapter Three, alcohol is 'The Best of All Medicines . . .' *up to a point.* 'Drink in moderation and live a longer life' does not apply to absolutely everyone. Therefore, I have deliberately tried to put forward a case for the harmful side of alcohol as well, rather than simply tell you which methods of drinking are most healthy. If you have certain predispositions or medical conditions, alcohol can actually make things worse. Some readers might even be put off drinking after reading this book.

As for me, writing this book led me to change my own drinking habits. I used to have a customary drink of an evening, but now I have stopped drinking at home if I am going out a lot during the week. I have upped the number of days that I give my liver a rest. Stepping on the scales, every morning and evening, is now a part of my daily routine. In other words, I still drink, but I also try to look after myself.

As ever, whenever I go out drinking, I exceed the recommended 'moderate amount', but with this new regime of care, my weight has gone down by three kilos, and my body fat has reduced by 5 per cent. I'm still on a diet . . .

My triglyceride levels, once over the standard value, are now within a nominal range. I wake up feeling refreshed and no longer have any bloating; both my body and skin condition are excellent. These results made me realise that the doctors' advice was truly correct. If I'd kept drinking as I had before, without any thought for the consequences, I could have deprived myself of work, and even work about drinking.

So, if you are an enthusiastic tippler, trust me and try the methods suggested in this book!

Of course, nothing will ever beat keeping to a 'moderate amount', but I know very well that it isn't as easy as it sounds. So, go on! Don't worry about it. It doesn't matter if you overindulge from time to time. Give the advice in this book a try. Your body will adapt, even if you are only 'aware of', rather than sticking to the moderate amount.

As you embark on your journey, if you find yourself feeling better than usual, then you've got it. Your body has naturally learned what a moderate amount should be, and you have developed a mode of drinking that doesn't give you a terrible feeling the morning after the night before.

This book also unravels a few mysteries, such as why water fills you up whereas you can drink so much more beer, and how we ever found the way home when we don't remember doing so. These are sure-fire topics for an entertaining and lively conversation at a table of drinkers, so do use it as a communication tool, too!

'Alcohol is not for drinking, but for tasting.'

Those are the words of the chairman of Asahi Shuzo Saké Brewing in Yamaguchi Prefecture, the maker of the famous Dassai drink. Rather than just drinking and getting drunk, I hope you will learn a mode of drinking that does not harm you, so that you can enjoy drinking, delicious food and delightful friends for the rest of your life.

Kaori Haishi, saké journalist

NHS Guidelines for Healthy Drinking

This book regularly gives one or two cups of saké, or a 500ml bottle of beer, as a daily limit for moderate drinking. As there are 180ml in a single *gō*, or cup, of saké and saké is generally 15 to 16 per cent ABV (alcohol by volume), this equates to between 5.4 and 5.76 units per day. A 500ml bottle of 5.2 per cent ABV beer equates to 2.6 units. The UK's National Health Service (NHS) guidelines suggest that men and women drink no more than fourteen units a week (six pints of average-strength beer or ten small glasses of low-strength wine) on a regular basis. *The Japanese Guide to Healthy Drinking*'s suggested limit is more permissive: between 18.2 and 40.32 units a week.

A standard glass of wine contains 175ml, while a large glass contains 250ml, or a third of a bottle. The ABV of wine generally ranges from 11 to 13 per cent, though sometimes this is lower, sometimes higher. Red wine generally has a higher ABV than white wine.

There is one unit of alcohol in a single measure (25ml) of spirits – gin, vodka, whisky, rum etc. – which tend to be 40 per cent ABV. There are two units in a double measure (50ml).

Everyday saké is 15–16 per cent ABV and cup of saké contains 180ml, which is the equivalent of 2.7 to 2.88 units. Undiluted saké (*genshu*) is 20 pe cent ABV, so a 180ml cup of this would be 3.6 units. You can work out how many units there are in any drink by multiplying the total volume of a drink (in millilitres) by its ABV and dividing the result by 1,000. So, a pint (568ml) of 5.2 per cent ABV beer is 2.95 units.

Type of drink	Number of alcohol units
Single small shot of spirits * (25ml, ABV 40 per cent)	1 unit
Alcopop (275ml, ABV 5.5 per cent)	1.5 units
Small glass of red/white/rosé wine (125ml, ABV 12 per cent)	1.5 units
Bottle of lager/beer/cider (330ml, ABV 5 per cent)	1.7 units
Can of lager/beer/cider (440ml, ABV 5.5 per cent)	2 units
Pint of lower-strength lager/beer/cider (ABV 3.6 per cent)	2 units
Standard glass of red/white/rosé wine (175ml, ABV 12 per cent)	2.1 units
Pint of higher-strength lager/beer/cider (ABV 5.2 per cent)	3 units
Large glass of red/white/rosé wine (250ml, ABV 12 per cent)	3 units

*Gin, rum, vodka, whisky, tequila, sambuca. Large (35ml) single measures of spirits are 1.4 units.

Source: www.nhs.uk/live-well/alcohol-support/calculating-alcohol-units/

All Drinkers Should Know the 'Right' Way to Drink

Oiled Up – how greasy foods reduce ill effects

Expert Adviser: Masashi Matsushima
Tōkai University School of Medicine

'The real drinkers[1] drink with salt as an accompaniment.'

That's a saying from Japanese olden times, and I often think it's true.

Most heavy drinkers stop eating when they start drinking. In fact, I am one of them. I get so absorbed in the drinking part that my consumption of food dramatically reduces, even though I know it will make me feel ill. And it only follows that drink-focused occasions with hardly any food on offer will often lead to severe sickness and nausea.

But when I drink with a proper food accompaniment, I hardly feel any discomfort at all, and my body condition cannot be better. 'Salt as an accompaniment' sounds pretty awesome and cool, but my experience tells me that it can't be good for your body. In fact,

---

1 The original text refers throughout to 'lefties' – *nomite*. In old-time Japan, the left hand was called the 'chisel hand' (*nomite*), because that's where a carpenter held his chisel. Since this sounds the same as 'drinker' (*nomite*) in Japanese, it's become a common term in drinking slang, but in English has the unfortunate side-effect of making every sentence sound like a political tract, or if rendered as 'chiseller', like a guide for masons. We have replaced the term throughout with 'drinker'.

I'm sure that quite a few readers will have suffered after drinking on an empty stomach.

So, what should we eat to avoid adverse effects? And when? We know we really should eat something, but what, exactly? Some people swear by drinking milk beforehand, but is that really effective?

I put these questions to Masashi Matsushima from the Tōkai University School of Medicine, a man with in-depth knowledge of the workings of the digestive system, including the stomach and intestines.

Blood alcohol content is the key

Even for those who don't think of themselves as heavy drinkers, it is important to know what kind of food you should eat either beforehand or at the beginning of a drinking session, in order to prevent intoxication. A friend of mine says: 'I love alcohol, but it doesn't like me. So, I have to drink milk or take a supplement beforehand.' Japanese people have a tendency to buckle under peer pressure and quite a few of them make an effort to force themselves to drink alcohol at parties.

'If you want to prevent hangovers and sickness,' says Professor Matsushima, 'you need to make sure that you don't let your blood alcohol content shoot up. If you have a high blood alcohol concentration, then you will become intoxicated, and there will be adverse affects. If you're not a strong drinker, it's what makes you feel sick or get tipsy. When the blood alcohol concentration increases still further, you may vomit or be unable to stand.'

So, what can we do to slow down the increase in blood alcohol concentration?

'The first organ to absorb alcohol in our body is the stomach. However, that only accounts for 5 per cent of all alcohol absorption.

The remaining 95 per cent is absorbed through the small intestine. There are outgrowths called *villi* on the lining of the small intestine, tens of millions in an adult body. The total surface area is said to be about the same as the area of a tennis court for an average adult male. Therefore, the small intestine has a much larger active area than the stomach, and it absorbs more alcohol with greater speed.

Blood alcohol concentration and drunkenness

	Blood alcohol concentration	Amount of alcohol	State of drunkenness
Sobriety	0.02–0.04%	- Beer 500ml bottle (up to one bottle) - Saké (up to 1 *gō*)	- Feeling exhilarated. - Face turns red. - Becoming cheerful.
Euphoria	0.05–0.10%	- Beer 500ml bottle (one to two bottles) - Saké (one to two *gō*)	- Slight intoxication. - Irrational behaviour. - Raised body temperature.
Excitement	0.11–0.15%	- Beer 500ml bottle (three bottles) - Saké (three *gō*)	- Becoming bolder. - Shouting. - Lack of balance when standing.
Confusion	0.16–0.30%	- Beer 500ml bottle (four to six bottles) - Saké (four to six *gō*)	- Drunken staggering. - Repeating oneself. - Feeling sick, vomiting.
Stupor	0.31–0.40%	- Beer 500ml bottle (seven to ten bottles) - Saké (seven *gō* to one *shō*)	- Unable to stand. - Stupefied. - Does not make sense.
Coma	0.41–0.50%	- Beer 500ml bottle (over ten bottles) - Saké (over one *shō*)	- Does not wake when shaken. - Becomes incontinent. - Risk of death.

one *gō* = 0.18 litre, one *shō* = 1.8 litre

Source: *Inshu no Kiso Chishiki [Basic Facts of Alcohol Consumption]* by the Health and Medicine of Alcohol Association

'Once alcohol reaches the intestines, it will get soaked up instantly. Therefore, the key to preventing the rise of blood alcohol content, which is to say, to delay getting drunk, involves keeping alcohol in our stomach for as long as possible, in order to delay it reaching the intestines.'

I see. So we need to keep the drink in the stomach for as long as possible to keep it away from the more efficient intestines.

'We call the period during which food is digested from the stomach and then expelled from it the gastric retention time,' says Professor Matsushima.

And the gastric retention time depends on the food that we have eaten. So, what kind of foods have a longer gastric retention?

At a drinking party, eat 'oily food' first

'That would be oil,' Professor Matsushima says. 'Oils have a longer absorption time in the stomach. With the help of CCK (cholecystokinin), a digestive hormone, it closes the pylorus, the exit from the stomach, and agitates the contents of the stomach.' (See the illustration on p.91)

What? Oil!? Sure, greasy food is heavy in the stomach and seems to have a longer gastric retention.

Gastric retention time differs from food to food. For example, while 100g of cooked rice will take 2 hours and 15 minutes to be digested, 100g of beef steak takes relatively longer, about 3 hours and 15 minutes. Oils have the longest retention times – 50g of butter, for example, can take up to 12 hours.

But even so, many of us would be hesitant to scoff greasy food merely to delay alcohol absorption.

'From the perspective of diminishing blood alcohol content, consuming oils beforehand makes sense,' says Professor Matsushima. 'But you don't have to just knock back oil in its raw form. There are many appetisers that have it as an ingredient, such as carpaccio, raw seafoods with olive oil, and potato salad with mayonnaise. I suggest you try something like that to start with, for their oil content.

'It might be a step too far as a starter, but fried chicken and chips would be just as effective. Any foodstuff that semi-solidifies when mixed with alcohol will take longer to reach the intestine.[2]

'Using snacks to create a situation that hinders the ability of the stomach and intestine to absorb alcohol is the key to maintaining a low blood alcohol content.'

Moreover, if you can't have oily food as a starter, there's always cheese, which contains lactic acid.

Milk and cabbage are good, too

What about drinking milk before alcohol? Is that effective?

'Milk has a fat content of just under 4 per cent, so you can expect an effect, to some extent. Its contents are protein-rich, which can offer some protection for the gastric mucosa. A small amount won't be enough to coat the whole stomach, but there should be some minor benefit.'

Professor Matsushima also mentions the effects of the enzyme S-Methylmethionine (SMM), which is sometimes nicknamed vitamin U.

'In addition to oils,' he says, 'it might be good at the beginning of a party to eat food with a high concentration of vitamin U, like cabbage.'

How does that help?

'Vitamin U in cabbages has a property of increasing the mucin on the mucous membranes within the stomach. Mucin is the main component of mucus discharged from the membrane, protecting the mucosa and stopping germs from getting through. A thicker layer of mucin increases the protective power of the mucous membrane, thereby guarding the stomach from alcoholic

---

2 Eating fatty snacks are good to start with, but make sure you don't eat too much, as they have a high calorie content.

stimulation. Although it has a marginal effect, it can still delay the speed of alcohol absorption. Tests on rats have shown that the effect of vitamin U starts to appear about one hour after eating.'

Come to think of it, yakitori restaurants in Japan, and places that sell deep-fried meat and vegetables on skewers (*kushiage*) do sometimes serve a starter comprising raw cabbage alongside miso or mayonnaise, so that makes sense, now.

Vitamin U, incidentally, is not actually a formally recognised vitamin, but it is naturally occurring in cabbage juice, and well known to maintain stomach health – in Japan there is even a gastrointestinal drug called Cabagin. If you want the best effects, cabbage is best eaten in its near-raw state, as vitamin U is water soluble and affected by heat. Cabbage fills your stomach, suppresses the appetite and is good for hydration, but be careful not to use too much salad dressing.

Other vegetables rich in vitamin U include broccoli and asparagus, so they are good, too. Professor Matsushima also recommends sticky, slimy foods such as beans, yams and okra.

Take taurine and sesamin to prevent adverse effects

So far, we've identified the foods that can delay drunkenness by slowing the onset of a higher blood alcohol content. But is there anything we can do to bring down the blood alcohol content while drinking, in order to prevent sickness and hangover?

Professor Matsushita says that this calls for supplementing the necessary metabolites required to break down alcohol.

'Once you've raised your blood alcohol content,' he says, 'it won't come down quickly. However, it would help to consume ingredients that would help the liver metabolise the alcohol more quickly – for example, taurine, found in octopuses and squids, L-cysteine, found in sunflower seeds and soy beans, and sesamin, which can be found in sesame seeds.

'It should go without saying that hydration is crucial. Alcohol has a diuretic effect, which means it increases the volume of urine, which can easily lead to dehydration. In order to prevent this, you should take fluids not only after drinking, but *while you are drinking*. After drinking, it is most effective to consume fluids that contain electrolytes, which aid water retention in the body.'

So, giving some thought to what you are nibbling on, before, during and after a drinking session can help prevent the kind of hangover that makes you never want to see a drink again.

However, any individual will have a limit in their abilities to break down alcohol, and once across that threshold, you will be sure to get a hangover, regardless of how carefully you've been choosing your bar snacks. Avoid excessive drinking!

The Morning After – how to avoid a rough hangover

Expert Adviser: Shinichi Asabe
Jichi Medical University Saitama Medical Center

A hangover is a state of ill health caused by alcohol or alcoholic metabolites, left in the body from the previous day's drinking. The symptoms can vary from headaches to nausea. The best way to avoid a hangover is simply not to drink too much. Many of us understand that, but once we're intoxicated, we can forget our self-control. We desperately want to avoid a rough hangover, so let us proceed with preventative measures.

'The basic cause of hangovers,' says Shinichi Asabe, a liver specialist at the Jichi Medical University Saitama Medical Center, 'is consuming alcohol in excess of your body's capacity to process it. To avoid that, you need to know what your personal limit for a moderate amount is.'

Mixing drinks risks losing sight of the amount of alcohol you have consumed

'It's especially dangerous to mix different types of alcohol,' he continues. 'It's because if you drink many different drinks, each with varying percentages of alcohol, you can risk losing sight of the total amount you have drunk.

'For example, you might start with a beer, and entering into the spirit of the party, move on to saké, and close with whisky on the rocks or an authentic *shōchū*. In this admittedly extreme scenario, you have already consumed a considerable amount of alcohol by the time you've got to the saké. Then you're on to whisky, which has more than 40 per cent alcohol content by volume (ABV). There's no way that your liver's alcohol-processing capacity is going to keep up with that, even though people's individual capacities can vary widely. There used to be a custom, which has now become a little outmoded, of making people at welcome parties chug a drink down in one go, and that's out of the question.

'When you down a drink in one go, you risk drinking enough to overload your alcohol processing capacity in a short period of time. The liver is unable to maintain its alcohol processing function, which leads to an accumulation of alcohol and aldehyde – a substance created in the process of metabolising alcohol. As a result, in the worst-case scenario, you could fall into a coma or even die.'

If you're in that situation, you are way over the threshold for a mere hangover. So how long does it take for the liver to process alcohol?

In order to come up with a number, we need to know the pure alcohol content. This is the amount of ethanol contained in the drink, which you can work out with this equation.

Alcohol content ÷ 100
× amount drunk in ml
× 0.8 (the specific gravity of ethanol)

Meanwhile, the amount of pure alcohol that a liver can process is roughly:
Bodyweight × 0.1

This is because the size of your liver is believed to be in proportion to your body weight. So if we have a person who weighs 100kg, the amount of pure alcohol they can process in an hour is 10g. Converted into alcoholic drinks, that is half of the average 500ml bottle of beer or a single shot of whisky, which is not much. For this reason, the first step for self-care is becoming aware of what the appropriate amount of drink is for yourself.

Formula to calculate the pure alcohol amount

ABV

÷   100 × the amount you have drunk (ml)

× 0.8 (the specific gravity of ethanol)

= Pure Alcohol Amount (amount of ethanol)

If you have consumed multiple types of drinks, you should add each of them to find the approximate value.

Put something in your stomach before drinking

'If you drink on an empty stomach,' says Dr Asabe, 'the alcohol will be quickly absorbed by your digestive organs, which increases the risk of a hangover. To prevent this, it's best if you eat something beforehand. If there is even a small amount of food in your stomach, the speed of alcohol absorption will be reduced, and that can prevent a hangover.'

According to Dr Asabe, the best type of food to eat beforehand is cheese. The protein and fat contained in cheese make it hard to absorb, so it lingers in the stomach, making alcohol absorption more gradual.

'Having solid food in your stomach gives you a sense of fullness,' he adds, 'which can encourage a slower drinking pace.' For a booze lover, the moment that beer pours into an empty stomach can be an instant of bliss, but if you want to prevent a hangover, you should get into the habit of eating before drinking.

Protein-rich *nattō* can protect the stomach

As we have seen, we should take care choosing the snacks we nibble on while we drink. You might tend to choose what's in season, or what the bar or restaurant recommends, but get into the habit of choosing instead on the basis of which components can help you ease a potential hangover. According to Dr Asabe, the elements you should actively consume are: protein, vitamin B1 and dietary fibre.

Protein

Once inside your body, protein will be broken down into amino acids and absorbed in the small intestine, which then carries it to the liver. Amino acids have the property of improving liver functions, which include detoxification and accelerating the metabolising of alcohol. You can consume animal-based protein, such as pork, beef or chicken, but if you are also watching your weight and counting the calories, you should choose a plant-based protein such as soybeans. Dr Asabe particularly recommends *nattō* – Japanese fermented beans.

'*Nattō* is protein-rich,' he says, 'but in addition, its uniquely sticky, slimy composition helps protect the gastric mucosa. It lessens the discomfort you might feel in your stomach the day after a drinking session.'

Vitamin B1

The second component on the list is vital in preventing alcohol and carbohydrates remaining in the body: the vitamin B group, and especially the crucial vitamin B1.

'When alcohol is broken down in the body,' he says, 'it's vitamin B1 that is consumed in large amounts. Vitamin B1 is an indispensable nutrient that helps metabolise carbohydrates and create energy. If your vitamin B1 levels drop because of a high intake of alcohol, you end up with a greater sense of fatigue the following day. It's a nutrient that you want to consciously ingest, not only during a drinking session, but also afterwards.'

Foods rich in vitamin B1 include pork, eel and cod roe. To help its absorption, the most effective combination is thought to be eating them with allicin, the main compound that creates the aroma and bitterness of garlic and onions.

Dietary fibre

And we mustn't forget dietary fibre. 'Dietary fibre reaches the colon without getting absorbed,' says Dr Asabe. 'Just like cheese, it stays within the digestive system for a long time, slowing down alcohol absorption.' To get a suitable hit of dietary fibre, it can be helpful to eat a small bowl of salad or boiled vegetables in a *dashi* sauce, before touching your first drink.

A lot of traditional Japanese 'taste of home' nibbles are rich in dietary fibre, such as *kinpira* – carrot and burdock or dried mouli and carrot in a sweet and savoury sauce. Actively seek out such a simple dish.

Hydrate often while drinking

In addition, Dr Asabe suggests we should drink water all through the session.

'Drinking water dilutes the alcohol concentration within the digestive organs,' he explains. 'We tend to get dehydrated after alcohol ingestion, because of its diuretic effects. So, in order to prevent that, it is best to start drinking water while enjoying the alcoholic drinks.'

As a case in point, the Japan Saké and Shōchū Makers Association (JSS) recommends drinking water between each sip of saké. It says that ideally you should drink as much water as you do alcohol. There's always some drunkard who brags that he'll 'drink beer as a chaser', but alcohol on top of alcohol will only accelerate dehydration.

We've explored a number of hangover prevention methods so far, but none of them amount to a hangover prevention *guarantee*.

Says Dr Asabe: 'The way to prevent a hangover is to keep eating balanced snacks that are rich in protein, fat, dietary fibre and vitamin B1. You should start drinking slowly, and drink in accordance with your assessment of your condition on that particular day.

'Drinking with food is a basic set-up, but many of us put our chopsticks down for good once the drinking begins. Alcohol is not for drinking, but for tasting, along with delicious food. If you keep that in mind, it should considerably reduce the risk of hangover.'

For Saké's Sake – improving your life with Japanese booze

Expert Adviser: Yukio Takizawa
Professor Emeritus at Akita University

Japanese saké is enjoying an unprecedented boom. Pure-rice saké (*junmai-shu*)[3] and *junmai ginjō-shu*[4] are particularly popular, with the quantity of production increasing from 109.4 to 120.1 per cent[5] year-on-year. Some famous brands such as Shinsei (from Akita Prefecture) and Jūyondai (from Yamagata Prefecture) are becoming difficult to find. The popularity is so great that there are saké events held all over Japan on most weekends.

I have been hosting and running saké events for a long time, but this upsurge is nothing like what I've seen in previous years. There are more female drinkers, and over half of the guests at the 'Saké 1 Grand Prix' event turned out to be ladies.

---

3 Translators' note – *Junmai-shu* is made only from rice, *koji*, and water, highlighting the flavour of the rice and *koji* more than other varieties. It is typically high in acidity and umami flavours, with relatively little sweetness (source: JSS). *Koji*, by the way, is a fungal fermentation culture, *Aspergillus oryzae*, used in the manufacture of soy sauce, bean pastes and various grain alcohols.

4 Translators' note – *junmai ginjō-shu* is a better grade than *junmai-shu*. The acidity and umami flavours are toned down, and it has a characteristic aroma and flavour (source: JSS).

5 Data from the National Tax Administration Agency, 2014 Sake production year.

If women are leading the trend now, we can expect saké to flourish even more. But when it comes to its effects on health, we are in a serious situation. Should we be treating saké as the villain? Many people believe that saké contains a lot of carbohydrates, so that people with diabetes or high blood pressure would be better off drinking authentic *shōchū* – a stronger, distilled grain alcohol. Some have even said they are doing so on their doctor's advice.

Stories like this are circulating and taken at face value, which makes me anxious as a regular saké drinker. More than anything else, it breaks my heart to see saké treated like it's the bad guy.

So, is saké good or bad for your health? To find out, I asked fellow saké lover Yukio Takizawa, a Professor Emeritus at Akita University. He's the author of several books, including *Two Gō a Day: How to Stay Healthy by Drinking Japanese Saké* (*Ichinichi Nigō: Nihonshu Iki-iki Kenkō-hō*, published by Kashiwa Shobō).

When I met him, the first thing I noticed was his beautiful skin. At eighty-four years of age, his skin was so smooth, and there were no traces of liver spots. There were no deep wrinkles carved into his skin, and his palms and inner arms were supple. I was lost in admiration. Professor Takizawa still drinks between 1.5 and 2 *gō* (360ml or less) a day. He must be a living exponent of the skin-enhancing properties of saké. Awesome . . .

The secret of saké's power is its rich amino acid content

But what about the health effect of saké? I didn't beat around the bush.

'Saké contains many nutritionally rich minor components,' Professor Takizawa assured me. 'Their indicated effects include anti-oxidant properties, inhibitors to blood coagulation, and anti-cancer effects, and they prevent lifestyle diseases. Drinking a moderate amount every day will have a positive effect on your health.'

'Saké contains more than 120 kinds of component nutrients, including amino acids, organic acids, and vitamins. In particular, saké's concentration of amino acids is far and away the best in any alcoholic drink. Indeed, these amino acids hold the key to saké's health properties, which do not exist in distilled beverages such as whisky or authentic *shōchū*.'

Amino acids have also been called the 'source of life'. Saké contains various kinds, with a good balance, including some essential amino acids that can't be produced within the body, such as lysine, tryptophan, leucine and isoleucine, as well as alanine, which supplies energy when we exercise. It also produces arginine, which helps regulate endocrine and cardiovascular functions and stimulates the secretion of growth hormones, as well as glutamic acid, which maintains immune functions and helps preserve the digestive tract. Notably, there's a large concentration of peptides – chains of amino acids – particularly in pure-rice saké, which, when created without additional brewer's alcohol, has a large quantity.

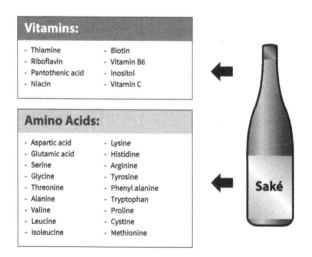

Vitamins:

- Thiamine
- Riboflavin
- Pantothenic acid
- Niacin
- Biotin
- Vitamin B6
- Inositol
- Vitamin C

Amino Acids:

- Aspartic acid
- Glutamic acid
- Serine
- Glycine
- Threonine
- Alanine
- Valine
- Leucine
- Isoleucine
- Lysine
- Histidine
- Arginine
- Tyrosine
- Phenyl alanine
- Tryptophan
- Proline
- Cystine
- Methionine

Saké

Saké is rich in amino acids. Its amino acid content is far greater than that of other alcoholic drinks, which contributes to its health benefits.

Peptide content in Saké

	Peptide content (mg/litre)
Junmaishu	6.89
Honjozoshu	6.12
General Saké	5.68

(Katsuhiko Kitamoto, et al., 1982)

The idea that diabetics can't drink saké is a thing of the past

'The biologically active peptides found in saké,' says Professor Takizawa, 'improve the susceptibility to insulin of a diabetic patient, and reduce the risks of heart diseases, such as high blood pressure and arteriosclerosis. The idea that diabetics can't drink saké is a thing of the past. Even the Japan Diabetes Society allows an intake of 1-gō a day (20g in pure alcoholic conversion), so long as glycemic control is fine and there are no complications. There is a theory that, apart from the peptides, the arginine in saké is also effective at combating diabetes.'

Diabetes, dubbed in Japan as the 'national disease', is an illness where a lack of insulin raises the glucose levels in the bloodstream, and the blood-sugar level remains high. Diabetics have to endure strict dietary restrictions, and saké, with high levels of carbohydrates, was regarded as 'bad'. It was a real surprise for me, and maybe even for you, that such a warning has now become outmoded!

Although the Japan Diabetes Society still only recommends a limited amount, this is surely good news for diabetics who have avoided saké. And it helps that the amino acids found in saké are, in Professor Takizawa's words, 'effective against lifestyle diseases in general'.

'Glutathione, a tripeptide comprising glutamic acid, cysteine and glycine, has an antioxidant effect, gets rid of the bad cholesterol that accumulates in blood vessels due to arteriosclerosis, and prevents ischemic heart conditions, such as angina and heart attacks. Cohort studies have already demonstrated this result, but as long as it is drunk in moderation, saké is likely to prevent lifestyle diseases such as diabetes.'

Saké can improve our ability to learn and memorise

As long as you keep to a moderate amount, saké can indeed be the best of all medicines. Moreover, its effect is likely to combat against various symptoms of ageing, starting with the memory disruption that can accompany ageing and senile dementia.

'A human being's learning function is carried out through the neural transmission of a hypothalamic hormone called vasopressin,' explains Professor Takizawa. 'When this neural transmission substance stops working normally, it causes memory disturbance. It is believed that this could be a root for the onset of senile dementia. Proline, one of the amino acids found in saké, is found throughout the human brain, and we know that it regulates the hormone vasopressin, improving our ability to learn and memorise.'

Apparently, the three peptides found in saké have been attracting attention in the Western world too.

Western Japan has more cases of cirrhosis and liver cancer

Professor Takizawa has published some interesting findings about the relationship between drinking alcohol, cirrhosis of the liver and liver cancer. Generally, it is believed that many cases of liver cancer and cirrhosis can be found among heavy drinkers. However, a regional diagram of mortality rates from these diseases in Japan shows a marked difference between east and west Japan – it's high in the west and low in the east, and this divide has been consistent since the end of the Second World War.

**Mortality rate for cirrhosis of the liver by prefecture
(standardised mortality ratio)**

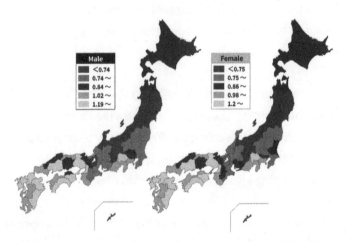

The standardised mortality ratio is a guideline used when comparing different age profile groups. The higher the figure, the higher the mortality rate. (Takizawa, et al., 1984)

The map shows a distribution diagram of the standardised death ratio from cirrhosis of the liver, by sex and prefecture, in a 1983 study that followed up an earlier survey in 1969 – notably, both were conducted before the medical establishment was aware of hepatitis C. A chart for liver cancer would show a similar distribution. The most popular alcoholic drink in western Japan is authentic *shōchū* (a distilled alcohol), whereas in the east it's saké (rice wine). 'There's a regional difference,' notes Professor Takizawa, 'in that both men and women consume more hard liquor in west Japan and rice wine in the east, and this has been true since at least 1945.[6] It's possible that this is a factor influencing the discrepancy in deaths, although there may have also been other variables.' It has been suggested that one

6 Translators' note – Professor Takizawa says *seishu* for 'rice wine' in the original Japanese, which is often interchangeable with *saké* in general conversation, but can sometimes refer to rice wine with an alcohol content of 22 per cent, slightly less than normal.

reason could be that western Japan, which is actually much further to the south, has a much higher infection rate of hepatitis C – a virus not even isolated and diagnosed until 1987. Carriers of hepatitis C are much more susceptible to harmful effects from drinking.

Saké suppresses cancer cell proliferation

Professor Takizawa has proved through testing[7] that minor components found within saké can have a suppressing effect on the proliferation of cancer cells. In his experiment, he introduced Akita pure-rice saké (undiluted, without heat treatment) into cultures containing human bladder cancer cells, prostate cancer cells and uterine cancer cells. Over the next 24 hours, saké with a 1:64 dilution factor caused 90 per cent of the cancer cells to die or undergo necrosis. Saké with a 1:128 dilution factor had a similar effect on 50 per cent of the cancer cells.

'I tried the same experiment with distilled spirits such as whisky and brandy,' he says, 'but the same effect could not be seen. The biggest difference between distilled spirits and fermented liquors like saké is the presence, or lack thereof, of the amino acids. Therefore, the effect is liable to be caused by the amino acids with a low molecular weight that we find in saké. Also, we know that it is a property of glucosamine, found in saké, that it can enhance the anti-cancer activity of natural killer cells.'

But what is a 'moderate' daily amount?

So, it looks like we can have a happy life if we keep drinking saké, with all its useful effects on diseases of modern society like cancer,

---

7 Takizawa, Y. et al., 'In vitro de saikin oyobi hito gansaibō no zōshoku wo sogaisuru seishu ni fukumareru inshi nitsuiteno kosatsu' [An in-Vitro Study of Factors contained in saké which impede proliferation of bacteria and human cancer cells], *Japanese Journal of Public Health*, 1994–06; 58(6): 437–440.

dementia and diabetes . . . but Professor Takizawa has a note of caution.

'That doesn't mean it's good to just drink without any care,' he says. 'The key is the *amount* that you consume. Too much is going to be bad.'

But how much is an ideal amount?

'The way to stay healthy is to keep to one or two *gō* of saké per day.' That's about 360ml or less, roughly two cups, or half the average 720ml saké bottle. 'For me, that means I don't have to give my liver a rest. Two *gō* a day is fine if you keep to that amount all week. Japan's Health and Medicine of Alcohol Association also recommends two *gō* as being a moderate amount.'

Professor Takizawa himself enjoys an uninterrupted nightly habit of one or two *gō* of pure-rice saké. But he says the key to enjoying saké's health benefits is 'to eat while drinking' and 'stop drinking when you are slightly tipsy'.

The benefits of saké have been claimed in Japanese medical texts since at least 1712, when they were cited in *Yōjōkun* (*The Book of Life-Nourishing Principles*) by Ekiken Kaibara. But more than enough is too much – do not overindulge!

The Incredible Shrinking Brain – should we worry?

Expert Adviser: Ryūsuke Kakigi
Professor at National Institute for Physiological Sciences,
National Institute of Natural Sciences

Forgetfulness is an everyday occurrence. You can't remember someone's name, momentarily forget how to spell a simple word, forget what you were about to do . . . It might be just a sign of old age for those of us who do not drink regularly, but for the drinkers, it can be a source of anxiety. We are bothered by the notion that too much drinking might be affecting our brain functions.

Does alcohol increase the risk of inducing brain diseases, such as subarachnoid haemorrhages, strokes and dementia? I put the question to Ryūsuke Kakigi from the National Institute for Physiological Sciences, National Institute of Natural Sciences.

Booze lovers' brains tend to shrink

'There are cerebrovascular risks,' he says, 'including cerebral infarctions triggered by lifestyle diseases, and alcoholism caused by routinely drinking to excess. The direct risk to the brain is believed to be reasonably low with moderate consumption, but if we examine the brains of frequent drinkers, we can see more shrinkage than average for their age, compared to those who do not drink very often.'

In other words, alcohol does shrink the brain!

Generally, brain shrinkage is an inevitable part of the ageing process, and tends to set in once we are in our thirties. Mainly, the shrinkage is called by the loss of the so-called white matter in the brain, which contains many nerve fibres. One of the subjective symptoms of brain shrinkage is the deterioration of memory, and if it progresses rapidly, it can cause dementia.

So the brain does shrink naturally as you get older, but Professor Kakigi has some concerns. 'Alcohol is believed to contribute substantially to the deterioration. If we compare MRI images from drinkers and non-drinkers of the same age, drinkers' brains tend to have 10 to 20 per cent more shrinkage than those of the non-drinkers. Notably, they tend to have enlarged lateral ventricles, which are the paired spaces, filled with fluid, in the cerebrum. This indicates that the lateral ventricles have expanded due to the shrinkage of the brain itself.'

So what parts of the brain are strongly affected by alcohol?

'In dementia and Alzheimer's, for example, these conditions are characteristically affected by the shrinkage of the hippocampus, which controls memory, the frontal lobe, which manages reasoning, and the anterior part of the temporal lobe, which covers language recognition, vision and hearing. But alcohol shrinks the *whole* brain. Recent research has shown a direct correlation between the amount of alcohol consumed and the amount of shrinkage in the brain, meaning that the longer your history of drinking, the more rapidly the brain is affected.

'Regardless of whether you have the odd day to give your liver a rest, or the kind of alcohol you drink (whether it's spirits or fermented liquors), your *lifetime* alcohol intake is believed to have a strong affect. Which means that the more you drink, the more your brain shrinks. The awful truth is that once neurons die in the brain, unlike stem cells in other organs, they will hardly ever regenerate or grow back to original size.'

He's got more bad news.

'Studies of men of an advanced age, who routinely drank a large amount of alcohol, indicate that their risk of succumbing to dementia was 4.6 times greater than men who drank less. Moreover, their risk of suffering depression was 3.7 times higher.'

There has yet to be a firm academic conclusion about the correlation between total lifetime alcohol consumption and the degree of shrinkage. However, the possibility is undeniable that excessive drinking increases the risk of some brain diseases.

You cannot 'train' your brain with alcohol

Even after they have learned that too much alcohol increases the risk of dementia and depression, many people cannot stay away from drinking. We can 'train' our liver to some extent by drinking, but I asked Professor Kakigi if we can induce a similar 'training effect' on our brains.

'Sadly, from a neuroscience perspective, I can't say that you can train your brain with alcohol like you can with your liver by upping the number of drinking occasions. If there was a way to do it, I would love to know, because I'm a bit of a drinker myself! As far as the brain is concerned, from a physiological point of view, alcohol is a poison right from the start.'

Brain shrinkage is part of the inevitable ageing process

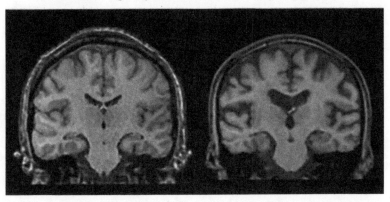

Twenty-five years old   Seventy-eight years old

These images compare the brains of two males, at twenty-five and seventy-eight years of age. We can see the lateral ventricle in the centre has grown bigger while the overall brain has become smaller. The brain is said to start shrinking after reaching a peak size at about thirty years old. About one hundred thousand nerve cells are said to die each day, and by the age of sixty or sixty-five, it becomes apparent from MRI scans that the brain has shrunk. Image: The Japan Foundation for Aging and Health, Kenkochoju Net, *Nō no Keitai no Henka [Change in Brain Shape]*.

I flinched at the notion he would go so far as to call it a poison, but make no mistake, many chemically composed medicines are also technically 'poisons'. There's that old Japanese saying we mentioned before: 'Saké is the best of all medicines.' So are there really no positive effects on the brain at all?

Let me bring in a graph that could provide a ray of hope. This is based on a study that investigated the correlation between alcohol intake and the risk of dementia, concluding that those who drink *moderately* (1–6 350ml bottles of beer a week) are at the lowest risk of developing dementia.

In short, there is a fine line between medicine and poison. There is a possibility that alcohol may still be the 'best of all medicines', even for the brain, as long as we get the dosage right.

Moderate drinking carries the
lowest risk of dementia

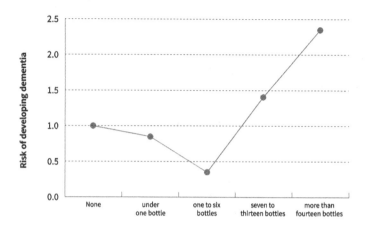

Amount of alcohol intake per week

This information is from a cohort study investigating alcohol consumption and the risk of dementia, conducted on 3660 men and women over sixty-five years of age in four regions in the US. The participants underwent MRI scanning and were re-checked from 1998 to 1999. The study revealed that when compared to abstention, a moderate consumption of one to six 350ml bottles of beer per week is associated with a lower risk of dementia. (Kenneth J. Mukamal, Lewis H. Kuller, Annette L. Fitzpatrick, et al 'Prospective Study of Alcohol Consumption and Risk of Dementia in Older Adults' in the *Journal of the American Medical Association*, Volume 289, Issue 11, March 19, 2003, 1405-1413.)

There is hardly any need to worry if you drink moderately

'It is true that alcohol shrinks the brain,' says Professor Kakigi, 'but unless there is a rapid change in the important areas within the brain, such as the hippocampus which controls memory, or the cerebellum that regulates balance, it's not going to affect your everyday life. There is hardly any need to worry, apart from a little bit of acceleration in brain shrinkage, as long as you stick to the rule of not drinking too much, and keeping to a moderate amount.'

Professor Kakigi, who calls himself a booze hound, suggested that measures against excess intake could include setting a time limit, after which someone from your family has to come and pick you up. If that's the situation, then you don't have the option to stay for just one more.

To stay healthy and enjoy drinking all through your life, hold onto a resolution to stop drinking as soon as you feel you want 'just one more'. That is indeed the way to drink without burdening your brain or your body.

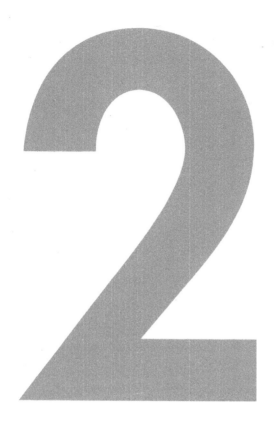

Self-Care – don't let alcohol win

Feel the Burn – the hidden dangers of karaoke

Expert Adviser: Toshiyuki Kusuyama
Tokyo Voice Clinic

Have you ever been out on a 'real session', drinking until late or even the early hours of the next morning, particularly during the holiday season at party after party . . . and then discovered the next day that your voice is hoarse, and that you have throat problems, including finding it hard to speak?

I'm sure I am not the only one to have noticed that a lot of long-term drinkers have a unique, raspy voice, like an experienced night-club hostess. Quite a few people believe that such a voice is caused by alcohol burn, or that the vocal cords have been damaged by alcohol.

Does alcohol burn really exist from a medical point of view? I asked Dr Toshiyuki Kusuyama, the head of otolaryngology at the Tokyo Voice Clinic Shinagawa.

Is smoking the cause of so-called 'alcohol burn'?

'For a long time, people have called that post-drinking raspy voice the "alcohol burn",' says Dr Kusuyama, 'probably because if you drink a high-ABV beverage like whisky, you get a sizzling sensation on the back of your throat. But, in fact, alcohol has no direct effect on the vocal cords. What *does* have a direct effect, on many of the patients who visit our clinic, is smoking.'

What a surprise: the commonly discussed 'alcohol burn' phenomenon turns out not to exist! But now that we know that cigarettes are the true cause of the hoarse voice, what exactly about the cigarette is doing the damage?

'Your vocal cords are located in a place called the larynx, between the epiglottis and the trachea. Your voice is generated by exhaled air, which turns into sound when the vocal cords close on either side, causing the membranes to vibrate. However, smoking causes the blood vessels in the vocal cords to constrict, interrupting blood circulation. On top of that, you get a low-temperature burn, which causes the vocal cords to swell or deform. If you think of them as being like a stringed instrument, if the strings swell or sag in places, the sound becomes raspy. Smoking also contributes to dryness, creating the worst possible environment for the throat.'

Most smokers smoke more cigarettes when they are drinking. If there's only temporary discomfort, there's no need to worry, but Dr Kusuyama has a warning.

'If you are a heavy smoker, and the swelling in the vocal cords becomes chronic, that will increase the risk of polypoid degeneration – blister-like disfigurements on both vocal cords.'

Looking at the Brinkman Index, which tracks the correlation between health and smoking, the risk of polyps increases dramatically with 'ten (per day) × twenty years'. This is higher than the risk of inducing laryngeal cancer, which is 'twenty (per day) × twenty years'.

The symptoms of polypoid degeneration include a hoarse or deep voice. If it is mild, the condition will improve simply through stopping smoking, but if it gets more serious, it may be necessary to perform surgery to remove the blistered cell tissues under the vocal cord mucosa.

Non-smoking is a must if you want to keep your voice beautiful. Needless to say, smoking is all pain, no gain, not only to your own throat, but to those non-smokers nearby who might suffer the effects of passive smoking. You'd better watch out for the condition of your throat and your voice.

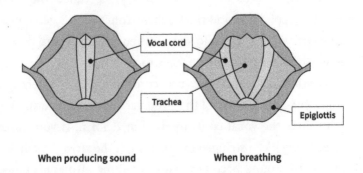

When producing sound   **When breathing**

The voice is created when the two vocal cords close on either side and the membranes vibrate. A deeper voice or hoarse voice is caused by the vocal cords not vibrating smoothly due to smoking, dehydration or age.

Acid reflux can also damage the vocal cords

However, even after our throat expert has concluded that a raspy voice is caused by smoking, that doesn't explain why non-smokers can still become hoarse after drinking. I hear all the time from my non-smoking drinker friends that they've lost their voice after a night of heavy drinking, they have trouble talking, or they have raspy voice. Is there really no causal relationship between alcohol and throat troubles?

'It's not so much directly caused by alcohol itself,' he explains, 'as other issues that might lead to a hoarse voice. For example, routine drinking can lead to acid reflux (an oesophageal mucosal injury caused by strong gastric acid and digested food travelling up towards the throat). Alcohol blunts the movement of the muscles that would usually stop the contents of the stomach from flowing back up. It increases the secretion of gastric acid, and that can injure the mucous membranes, as well as imparting an adverse effect on the vocal cords.'

Come to think of it, that sour taste of gastric acid is more frequent after drinking... I didn't realise that acid reflux affects not only stomach and the oesophagus but also the voice.

'A second possible cause is dehydration in your body caused by drinking,' says Dr Kusuyama. 'Alcohol suppresses the antidiuretic hormone (ADH), resulting in an increased discharge of urine, which can lead in turn to dehydration and dryness of the throat. Alcohol in the blood vessels can deprive the cells of moisture. Vocal cords vibrate 200–250 times a second in women and 100–120 times for men, but dryness can impair that smoothness of the movement, and cause trouble for the voice. Dryness is also the cause of a hoarse voice from too much talking. And incidentally, too much salt intake from snacks will also swell the vocal cords, and cause you to lose your voice.'

You might find Dr Kusuyama's explanation convincing enough on its own, but apparently there is an even worse danger, and that is karaoke after drinking. If you are a drinker who loves singing, you can't ignore this issue. Many of you might be looking forward to venting a year's worth of pent-up feelings at a karaoke bar, maybe even the second or third venue of the night.

The absolute worst: post-drinks karaoke with added dancing

'Karaoke after drinking combines the three biggest risks to the vocal cords,' says Dr Kusuyama. 'First of all, if you force yourself to sing in a higher key than your natural voice, it places the vocal cords under stress. Secondly, if you are going to sing and dance along, additional motion increases respiratory volume. If you're singing loudly on top of it, the vocal cords suffer double damage and risk of dryness. You try to moisten your throat with another alcoholic drink, and that just increases the ADH and dehydrates your body. And then you are talking in a loud voice. You place a burden on your vocal cords by having to speak up in a noisy environment. When you are chatting, you tend to breathe more through your mouth, which also dries out the vocal chords. And incidentally, oral respiration requires six times the effort of nasal respiration.'

So, you're singing golden oldies with your super dance moves, or bopping together when the party gets underway. It's not uncommon for other people to join in with the singer . . . Apparently, many aerobics instructors, whose job involves constant bodily motion while yelling instructions, suffer from conditions such as vocal nodules – vocal cords damaged from the double burden of exercise and vocalisation.

But if you start to worry about a hoarse voice after drinking, is there any way you can prevent the deterioration?

If you have a hoarse voice for longer than one month, get an endoscopy

'Unfortunately, you cannot "train" your vocal cords,' says Dr Kusuyama. 'The cellular water-retention capacity of our body decreases with age, so getting a deeper voice is inevitable to a certain extent. In that regard, the best way to prevent dehydration is to drink moderately. If you are drinking alcohol, drink water as often as possible. This will increase the secretion of airway mucus, which can protect the vocal cords from drying out. If you have to go to parties day after day, try not to raise your voice, and control your alcohol intake. If you have problem talking for more than month, I recommend you go to see an ear, nose and throat specialist, and have an endoscopic examination.'

I am sure that a hoarse voice would affect many people's job performance. Now we know that so-called alcohol burn doesn't exist, and that the best remedy is to steel yourself not to be the one who goes out partying every night and then says: 'Now, let's go to karaoke!'

Mellow Yellow – checking the colour of your pee

Expert Adviser: Matsuhiko Hayashi
Keiō University Hospital

Once you've got a few glasses into a drinking session, your main desire is to urinate. But once you start going to the loo, you find yourself visiting it more often than expected in a short period of time, as if a dam has suddenly broken. While many drinkers tend to regard this physiological phenomenon favourably as a chance to get rid of some alcohol from the body, there can be a hidden danger. The potential disaster area is the kidneys.

I asked Matsuhiko Hayashi, a professor at Keiō University Hospital, about the correlation between alcohol and the kidneys, organs with important functions that include creating urine and excreting waste matter from the blood.

The volume of urine can be as much as 1.5 times your alcohol intake!

'There's a reason why you have to go to the toilet frequently when drinking,' says Professor Hayashi, 'and that's the suppression of the antidiuretic hormone (ADH) located in the pituitary gland. As a result you release more urine than necessary. In fact, the amount of urine discharged can be 1.5 times what you actually drank. Far from rehydrating, intake of alcohol, including beer, can reduce the water content in the body, which can cause dehydration.'

There are many drinkers who use beer instead of water as a chaser, but that does not help their rehydration at all. I am sure many readers have had the experience of getting thirstier as they drink more. But can't we just drink more water to supplement the moisture lost due to alcohol?

'Sure, you should drink water,' he says, 'but the question is the amount. Drinking too much water can harm the body. Excessive water intake will dilute the sodium concentration in your blood more than necessary, causing hyponatremia, with symptoms such as despondency, loss of appetite, and nausea. The best option is to ingest roughly the same amount of water as alcoholic drinks.'

According to Professor Hayashi, there are guidelines we can use for preventing adverse effects from drinking. One of them is the change in urine colour.

Darker and decreased output is a sign of dehydration!?

The usual colour of urine in a healthy person is light yellow. The pigment that makes the yellow colour is a substance called urobilin. This is a by-product of the degradation of haem – one of the components of blood haemoglobin.

'In other words,' says Professor Hayashi, 'if your urine is light yellow, it contains a moderate amount of urobilin, and there isn't too much water. If you drink too much water, the colour becomes paler and more translucent. On the other hand, if you're drinking alcohol without hydration, the liver cannot work as well as it should, there is less water and comparatively more urobilin, so the colour of the urine looks darker. Moreover, if there is less urine than normal, then it is an indicator that you are becoming dehydrated.'

So, far from being pleased with yourself, that frequent toilet trips are purging your body of alcohol. In fact they are purging your body of *water*, and if the amount you urinate decreases, your body may be running out of it!

We tend to think of the kidney's function as one of simply detoxing and creating urine, but it plays an important role in the regulation of the body's water retention. Additionally, the kidney controls the body's vital levels of sodium.

'For example, if we consume too much salt, that will naturally increase the level of sodium concentration in the blood. As a result, the osmotic pressure will increase inside the cells, to increase moisture. When that happens, the brain secretes a hormone to the kidneys, which orders them to bring the sodium concentration back up to a normal level of around 0.9 per cent. This is the reason why we get thirsty, because we want to drink water.'

But if that's the case, watch out for the snacks you eat alongside your drinks.

Bars *want* you to be thirsty, so they favour bar snacks with salt in them – a 28g serving of roasted salted peanuts contains 119mg of salt. But if we look at the kind of bar snacks offered to Japanese drinkers, the salt content is much higher – three fried *satsuma-age* fishcakes contain 3.3g of salt; five or six dried fat sardines (*maruboshi*) have about 2.0g; and three pieces of *kara-age* fried chicken will have 1.16g. Worst of all, *shiokara*, a kind of salty fish paste, racks up 4.8g of salt per serving.[8]

Compare that to the recommended practical daily intake of sodium, as set by the Japanese Ministry of Health, Labour and Welfare – less than 8g for men and 7g for women. If you snacked on just three or four servings of the items listed above, you would

8 Source: Kagawa Nutrition University, *80 Kilo Calorie Guide*.

go way over the figure. Even *oden*, a little hotpot that goes well with saké, has a high salt content, so watch out!

Alcohol will dehydrate your body enough on its own, but if you add a double-whammy of sodium, the spiral of thirst risks getting out of control. The body requires more and more water, but instead of water, the drinkers tend to reach for more alcohol to quench their thirst . . .

Simulation of renal function (GFR) decline

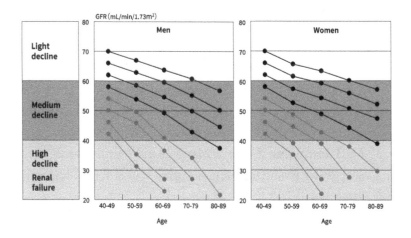

It is known that GRF, the indicator of renal function, declines by roughly 1 per cent every year from forty years of age. The black lines in the graph are a simulation of the decline using the value at forty years old as the base. The grey lines in the graph are when the person has chronic kidney disease (CKD). As the person gets older, the decline of renal function is predicted to deteriorate even more. Once GFR value drops below twenty, dialysis is required. (Japan Society of Nephrology, Committee of Measures for CKD, Epidemiology WG, 2006.)

Frequent urination is also a sign of age-related renal decline

'Bodily fluids are held in the kidney by the glomerulus, a tuft comprising about two million small blood vessels,' explains Professor Hayashi. 'They keep sodium concentration at the optimum level. Their functions include filtering blood from the heart, extracting glomerular filtrate, which is eventually expelled as urine. When glomerular function declines due to ageing, the capacity for water retention can decrease, and if that happens, the colour of urine can be paler. In other words, if you are discharging darker yellow urine, it means that waste matters are being properly excreted, so the kidney function is working well.'

Age-related deterioration varies depending on the individual and their gender, but the glomerulus filtration rate (GFR), will start to decrease at about 1 per cent a year once we hit our forties. Just thinking about it gives me the shivers. And Professor Hayashi warns that habitual drinking will decrease that capacity still further.

'When GFR goes down,' he says, 'the body begins to lose its ability to hold onto water, and that means that you need to urinate more frequently. That, in turn, means that as you get older, you are more easily dehydrated. On top of that, when alcohol is suppressing your ADH levels, you will discharge even more urine, losing more and more water from the body. It's much easier for middle-aged and old-aged drinkers to get dehydrated.'

That is why it's better to keep an eye on the colour of your urine when you are drinking, as well as drinking a moderate amount of water, all the better to prevent dehydration.

Is there any way you can bring your GFR back up?

'Unfortunately, no,' says Professor Hayashi. 'There isn't a way with current medical knowledge that can bring a GFR value up once kidney function undergoes a chronic decline.' You might see advertisements for supplements that claim to improve kidney functions every now and then, but so far, there is no definitive research data that proves their effectiveness.

If you have difficulties or concerns about your urine, you should consult with your doctor as soon as you can.

So, it seems that the only way to reduce the burden on the kidneys is to reduce your intake of alcohol and salt?

'As a specialist, yes,' says Professor Hayashi. 'Excessive ingestion of alcohol and salt will put a burden on your kidneys and liver, so I wouldn't recommend it. But if you can't stop yourself drinking altogether, you can still monitor the following factors: obesity, high blood pressure and smoking. Each of them has been proven to heighten the burden on our blood vessels, and to have a negative effect on GFR. In order to minimise the damage to your kidneys, you should take the same measures you would take against lifestyle illnesses.'

And those would be the kind of lifestyle illnesses most likely to affect a drinker. Those two little words, 'moderate amount', can be a high hurdle to clear. But if you care about your kidneys, try to make a little bit of effort.

Snack Attacks – secrets for avoiding weight gain

Expert Adviser: Hiroyuki Hayashi
Shibuya DS Clinic Shibuya

'I want to drink a lot, but don't want to put on weight.'

Obesity is a hazard that hovers at the back of the mind of many a drinker. Sure enough, looking at the habitual drinkers I know, I'd hesitate to call them slim. On the contrary, quite of a few of them are suffering from lifestyle illnesses such as fatty liver, diabetes or gout, all of which are said to be related to obesity.

Some recent diet fads have claimed that alcohol won't make you fat because it contains **empty calories** – it's not that the alcohol has no calories, but that the calories it contains are relatively low in nutrients. But that can't be true, because I certainly put on weight after a few drinking sessions in a row.

So, for starters, does alcohol itself accelerate weight gain?

I put the question to Hiroyuki Hayashi from Shibuya DS Clinic, a specialist weight-loss institution.

Alcohol alone would not give you much weight gain?

'Let's begin by discussing the alcohol content,' says Dr Hayashi. 'Pure alcohol is 7.1 kilocalories per gram, but we know that about 70 per cent is metabolised and consumed. This is one reason why people claim that alcohol has "empty calories", in the expectation that it won't make you put on weight. Compared with the same calorific intake from fats or carbohydrates, it has no nutritional value, so it has less effect on your gaining weight. So, in light of that, it's probably safe to say that pure alcohol alone will not make you put on weight. However, fermented liquors, like beer, saké or wine, contain things like carbohydrates and proteins, so drinking them certainly *will* increase your calorie intake. So, it's vital to keep to a moderate amount.'

When Dr Hayashi talks of a moderate amount, he's thinking of 20–40g in pure alcohol. Converted into saké, that would be a figure we have seen before, one or two *gō* (360ml or less). In fact, for those who want to lose weight but don't want to stop drinking, Dr Hayashi's clinic allows up to 200 kcal of alcohol daily, which is 350–500ml of beer, or just under three glasses of wine. Dr Hayashi, who openly admits to enjoying a drink himself, says: 'Personally, I make sure my alcohol intake is within 200 kilocalories, and I tend to choose low-sugar alcohol drinks that are purine-free.'

We eat too many snacks!

However, many people still manage to put on weight, even if they keep to the moderate amount. The reason is simple.

'They eat too many snacks with their alcohol,' points out Dr Hayashi.

Let's look at a typical menu that might be ordered at an *izakaya*, a Japanese pub.

- A medium glass of beer (350–500ml): 200 kcal
- Fried chicken (3 or 4 pieces, c.120g): 286 kcal
- Fried fishcake (2 pieces, c.100g): 150 kcal
- Potato salad (c.120g): 200 kcal

Tot all that up, and we've just had 836 kilocalories. But it's not like the average drinker is going to be happy after just one glass of beer. There are some who go on the 'drunkard's golden course', starting with a beer, then saké, wine, authentic *shōchū*, and then rounding it all off with a big bowl of ramen. And let's remember, ramen started out as a hearty workman's lunch that was supposed to be an entire meal in itself – if you're ordering *tonkotsu* ramen (pork bone soup), that will contain back fat, roast pork and hard-boiled eggs, and if you drink up the soup as well, you're going to notch up 2000 kcal.

So now we've just easily taken in 3000 kcal, with a 'drinking' session that started off with just one beer. If you stock up with high-calorie snacks late at night, it's no wonder if you gain weight, even if you are monitoring your alcohol consumption and trying to watch your weight.

Late makes weight

If you want to keep enjoying alcohol without gaining weight, it's best to get into the habit of watching your daily calorie intake while eating.

'For routine drinkers,' says Dr Hayashi, 'the key is to calculate the total calorie intake of the snacks. But there is a crucial point to bear in mind: eat three square meals and do not skip one. You can have a light breakfast and lunch, such as fruits in the morning and noodles at midday, but skipping breakfast and having a light lunch is a no-no. Because if you have an empty stomach all day, you are far more likely to eat a big meal in haste in the evening, which is liable to give you an increased calorie intake.'

In particular, he warns clients to be careful about starting drinking sessions too late, as that will help them avoid over-eating. He recommends starting the session by eating foods that are high in fibre and low in calories, such as salads or crudités. By doing so, you're leaving less space for high-calorie snacks later on. At the same time, you can expect them to shield the walls of your stomach and intestines from alcohol damage.

To further reduce the calorie intake from snacks, avoid greasy food and look out for food that is steamed, stewed, grilled or boiled. At a Japanese diner, you can look out for dishes like vegetables and seaweeds – *edamame*, tomatoes, seaweed or cucumbers marinated in vinegar, and low-fat high-quality, protein-rich dishes such as hot tofu, and *ikasomen* (fine raw squid strips). On the other hand, if you go for high-calorie, high-fat, high-carbohydrate snacks, such as savoury pancakes, pizza, dumplings, potato salad or fried chicken, you will increase your triglyceride levels, leading to weight gain. Drinking parties often involve rounds of salty, rich food to encourage more eating and drinking, and as a result, we eat and drink more than we anticipated.

Nine kilocalories makes one gram of fat

Dr Hayashi has advice to get you out of the vicious circle.

'Think of a few days as a single unit, and try to adjust the rhythm and cycle of meals within it.'

For busy businesspeople, a method that adjusts to a cycle that is several days long is relatively easy to tackle.

'First of all, set a "reference point" with your current body weight, and get into the habit of stepping on a scale every morning. If your weight is over the set range, avoid fats and carbs as much as you can, and take meals that are rich in vegetables and vegetable proteins. In order to keep drinking without gaining weight, it's critical that you get into the habit of not saving fat.'

If you spoil yourself by saying that it won't count if you gain just a kilo, then that's going to be a negative saving. If your body has nine kilocalories of unconsumed excess energy, it will be converted physiologically into 1g of fat.

It might sound like a tiny amount, but such trifles can add up if they continue day after day, and your body weight will definitely go up. To prevent that from happening, you need to control your calories, using your reference weight as a guide.

'If you really love drinking, and wish to keep drinking your whole life, you can do it,' says Dr Hayashi with a smile. But to avoid a downward spiral into weight gain and the lifestyle illnesses that come with it – deterioration of uric acid values, increase in triglycerides and rise in blood glucose levels – it's essential for a drinker to maintain a steady, daily and persistent effort.

Fear of a Fat Liver – pay attention to your medical results!

Expert Adviser: Shinichi Asabe
Jichi Medical University Saitama Medical Center

Many businesspeople worry about a fatty liver.

For many of us, it's the first thing we check when we get the results of our medical. And the name is very descriptive – when you hear the words 'fatty liver', you can easily picture that it's a disease which stems from obesity due to excessive intake of fats and carbohydrates. But perhaps because of the theory, debunked in the previous section, that alcohol can't make you fat because it only contains 'empty calories', you might be forgiven for thinking that alcohol has nothing to do with fatty liver, or even if it does, not so much – at least, I certainly believed that myself for a long while.

However, there is in fact a strong correlation. It has become clear that one of the causes of fatty liver is alcohol itself.

I think of my friends who like drinking, and there are far more of them who are overweight than thin. Even the ones who do look thin have often been diagnosed with high triglycerides, as being at-risk of getting a fatty liver, or actually having a fatty liver.

I myself am of average weight, but sadly my triglyceride levels are on the high side. I have not been diagnosed as officially overweight, but it's obvious to me that I am secretly obese.

When it comes to food, I do look after myself, mainly sticking to vegetables for my snacks, but why am I secretly obese? Is alcohol to blame?

Those of you who are deeply in love with alcohol must be sincerely hoping that you can carry on this affair for your whole life. But there must be many people, including me, who secretly worry themselves sick that if they keep going on the way they are, they will end up with a fatty liver.

I asked Shinichi Asabe from the Jichi Medical University Saitama Medical Center about the correlation between alcohol and fatty liver.

One in three Japanese people have fatty liver!?

'One in three Japanese people are said to suffer from a fatty liver,' he said. There is a report that 32 per cent of Japanese adults who had a medical turned out to have fatty liver. Another report noted that 58 per cent of those with light obesity (a body mass index of between 25 and 28) had fatty livers.[9]

When compared with similar results for Westerners, the data shows that liver morbidity among the Japanese is considerably high. What is this condition, which started to spread when we Japanese started adopting Western dining fads?

'Fatty liver disease is a condition where fats, especially triglycerides, start to build up in your liver,' explains Dr Asabe. 'To put it simply, it's similar to the way we make foie gras. The mechanism is very basic – if the amount of fat created exceeds the amount that the liver is putting out, then it stores the extra fat as "savings" and that causes the problem.'

We all like saving money . . . saving fat, not so much. However,

---

9 BMI (body mass index): a figure that tests the balance between weight and height.

how alarmed does someone get if they hear they have a fatty liver? Honestly, I think a lot of people think it's okay to just ignore it. But that would be a big mistake.

'Do not take a fatty liver lightly,' cautions Dr Asabe. 'If you ignore the condition and do not make changes to your lifestyle, you can develop inflammation, or develop fibrosis[10] that leads to a "hard liver", and in the end you can get cirrhosis of the liver or liver cancer. Because the liver has a strong capacity to regenerate, the progress can be slow. Therefore, there are quite a few cases where people only suddenly realise that their condition has deteriorated.'

One in three Japanese people have a fatty liver!?

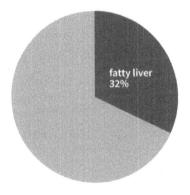

fatty liver
32%

The study said 32 per cent of Japanese adults who had a health check turned out to have a fatty liver. The chart shows the ratio of those with fatty liver from 1578 Japanese adults (1208 men, thirty-five to sixty-nine years old), who went for a check-up at a health centre. (Katsuhisa Omagari, Shunichi Morikawa, Seiko Nagaoka, et.al, 'Predictive Factors for the Development of Regression of Fatty Liver in Japanese Adults' in *Journal of Clinical Biochemistry and Nutrition*, Volume 45, Issue 1, July 2009, 56-67.)

---

10 Liver fibrosis: a chronic inflammation kills hepatocyte tissue, which allows fibrous tissue to proliferate. When the whole liver turns fibrous, this is hepatic cirrhosis (cirrhosis of the liver).

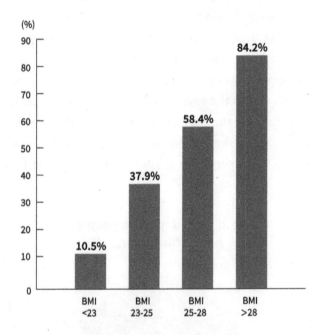

**The higher the degree of obesity,
the more the chances of a fatty liver**

This data examines the incidence rate of fatty liver disease per degree of obesity (BMI). We can see that the higher the degree of obesity, the greater the chance of getting fatty liver disease. (Eguchi, Y. et al., 'Prevalence and associated metabolic factors of non-alcoholic fatty liver disease in the general population from 2009 to 2010 in Japan: a multicentre large retrospective study' in *Journal of Gastroenterology*, Volume 47, Issue 5, February 11, 2012, 586-595.)

Alcohol is the direct cause of fatty liver

So we should never take a fatty liver lightly.

'Aside from a high-calorie diet and a chronic lack of exercise,' adds Dr Asabe, 'one of the causes of a fatty liver is alcohol itself.'

So far from 'not making you fat', alcohol is actually a direct cause of fatty liver. For booze lovers like me, this is an inconvenient truth that makes us want to scream.

'There are two types of fatty liver,' he says, 'alcoholic fatty liver disease, caused by excessive drinking, and non-alcoholic fatty liver disease, caused by obesity, dyslipidemia and diabetes. Generally, more patients present with non-alcoholic fatty liver disease, but if you are a heavy drinker, the risk of the alcoholic kind is high.'

Now that we know that alcohol can directly cause a fatty liver, the next question is how.

Fatty liver disease category

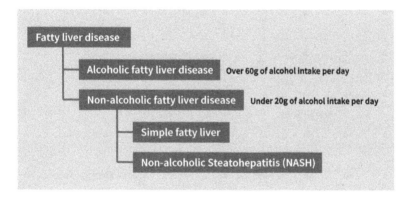

Fatty liver is a condition in which fat (especially triglycerides) builds up in the liver in the hepatic cells. Fatty liver disease is roughly divided into Alcoholic fatty liver disease and Non-alcoholic fatty liver disease. Non-alcoholic fatty liver disease is further divided into Simple fatty liver and Non-alcoholic Steatohepatitis (NASH).

Fat-burning is impeded by the metabolising of alcohol

According to Dr Asabe, there are two reasons why an excessive alcohol intake can lead to a fatty liver.

'Firstly, alcohol is a component in triglycerides. Alcohol dehydrogenases turn the ethanol delivered to the liver into acetaldehyde (ADH1B), and then aldehyde dehydrogenases turn that into acetic acid. After that, it turns into acetyl-CoA, and eventually it generates energy and creates fatty acids. This becomes the triglycerides.

The process of alcohol metabolism

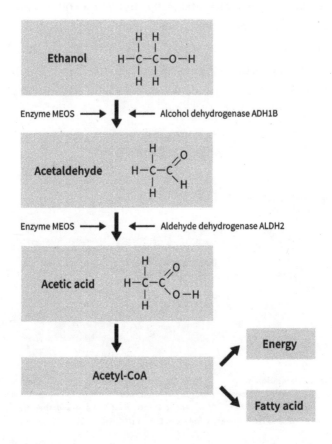

Approximately 90 per cent of alcohol (ethanol) is metabolised in the liver. Ethanol is turned into acetaldehyde and acetic acid before eventually becoming energy and fatty acid.

'But another reason is that during the metabolising of alcohol in the liver, fat-burning is impeded. Usually, our bodies use "beta-oxidation" to metabolise fatty acids. Beta-oxidation is a process that oxidises the fatty acids to ultimately generate the energy that our cells require. But when the liver metabolises alcohol, the beta-oxidation is suppressed, which interferes with the fat-burning, and causes excess, unmetabolised fatty acids to be stored in the liver. That's why fatty livers become an issue with people who like to drink.'

I see . . . so there is a direct cause between drinking too much and getting a fatty liver.

'When your pure alcohol intake per day is over sixty grams (three *gō* of saké, or about 540ml), you are most certainly going to be suffering from a fatty liver. The fact that excess alcohol leads to fatty liver is the commonest of common knowledge in medicine to be found in text books.'

But I didn't know this, even though it's 'common knowledge' . . .

Total alcohol intake is more important than a liver holiday

Since it's clear that alcoholic fatty liver disease is caused by drinking, you might think that you could just give your liver a rest for a few days, but Dr Asabe says differently. 'It's more important,' he says, 'to reduce your total alcohol intake than it is to give your liver a holiday.'

'A moderate amount is about 150g a week in pure alcohol conversion. It may be effective to have a day of rest for your liver, but that's no use if you go back to binge-drinking the day afterwards. If you want to improve the state of a fatty liver, it is better to focus on keeping the total amount of drinking under control.'

He adds that choices of snacks are important.

'You particularly need to watch out for too much carbohydrate intake. Alcohol suppresses the liver's ability to release glucose, so the blood-sugar level does not go up easily, and we get a feeling of emptiness in our stomach. So if we choose to satisfy that hunger with something that's heavy in carbs, like a savoury pancake or fried noodles, we get into a negative spiral which stores even more fat.'

So the metabolising of alcohol causes fat to accumulate, but if we add the fat from snacks on top of that, it's another double-whammy. The taste of ramen after a drinking session is wonderful, but don't be fooled by the false sense of hunger that alcohol can induce.

Fool your check-up, fool yourself

The advice, often repeated, has been to reduce alcohol intake and watch out for snacks, but are there are any other points we should bear in mind?

'Go for regular health checks,' says Dr Asabe. 'And most importantly of all, don't stop drinking just because there is a medical coming up. Health checks are completely useless unless they can evaluate your everyday lifestyle status. If you avoid drinking for the day and get a good result, that will only be temporary. To know the true capabilities of your liver, and to face up to the damage you might be doing to it at your habitual pace, I recommend that you *don't* alter your lifestyle just because a medical is coming up.'

The advice makes my ears burn, but he's right – the purpose of a medical is not to hack it into giving you a good score, but to get a true assessment of your current condition. If the result is disappointing, then maybe stop drinking for a month and go back for a second check-up. If the scores have not improved, then the cause could be something other than alcohol. In other words, don't take the temporary measure of avoiding alcohol before a medical, because you will then be able to check for 'hidden illnesses'.

According to Dr Asabe, you need to keep an eye on the following levels – the triglycerides (TG), the gamma-GTP that contributes to liver detoxification, and the ALT (GPT) that indicates how much liver tissue has been damaged. But if you know you have a fatty liver, it is best to get an ultrasound and CT scan along with the blood test, in order to get a fair diagnosis.

Probably because fatty liver cases are on the rise, there are many advertisements offering 'cures' for a fatty liver, but apparently liver supplements can actually make things worse. In particular, fat-soluble treatments like beta-carotene and vitamin E can accumulate in the body, so you should consult a doctor before taking them, rather than prescribing them for yourself.

The treatments that have been proved to work with fatty liver are diet and exercise. Moderate drinking, and moderate exercise, along with a balanced diet, are still the best medicine.

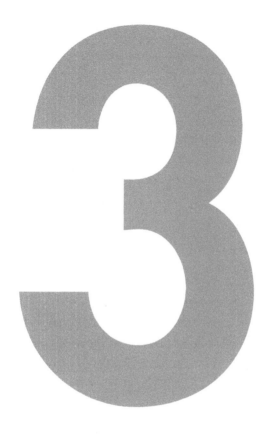

Staying Healthy – rules for avoiding drink-related illness

Our Survey Said – 140,000 people's advice on drinking and staying healthy

Expert Adviser: Shōichirō Tsugane
National Cancer Center

'You cannot drink alcohol if you are worried about getting ill!'

'Drink! Drink! Bring me a drink!' So many drinkers brag about it when they are overconfident, hot-blooded youths, and even now when they are little longer in the tooth. But as you get older, you simply can't drink at the same pace you maintained when you were younger. Lifestyle illnesses, like obesity and high blood pressure, will start to creep up on you. And the same problems can hound those who are forced to drink on business.

You might try to tough it out and tell me that a high level of uric acid and gamma-GTPs are some sort of badge of honour. But in the real world, illness is scary. So, I went to ask Shōichirō Tsugane from Japan's National Cancer Center about the correlation between alcohol and illness.

'Let's start by saying that alcohol is a poison for the body,' he says. 'If you keep drinking more than a moderate amount for a long time, of course the risk of developing an illness is going to increase. If we look at male alcohol intake, for example, the difference between a man drinking two cups a day of saké, and three cups or more a day is that the former is 1.4 times as likely, and the latter is 1.6 times as likely to get cancer as an occasional drinker who only has a cup of saké once or fewer times a week.

'As far as the location of the cancer goes, if you're drinking more than two cups of saké a day, you are 4.6 times more likely to get oesophageal cancer and 2.1 times more to get colorectal cancer. There's also research that indicates you are 1.4 times more likely to suffer a stroke.'

I don't like hearing that alcohol is poison, but how can I argue with those figures?

In which case, where do these numbers come from?

140,000 people can't be wrong . . . every few years

'The figures I'm quoting are from what we call a multi-purpose cohort study. That's when we take epidemiological observations over a long period of time. This was a large-scale project begun in 1990, tracking 140,420 people in eleven regions all over Japan. We looked for correlations within this set group, using statistics about their lifestyle, including drinking, diet, smoking and exercise, and how they affect the quality of life (QOL) and illness.'

Not everybody is familiar with cohort studies. But this one has generated scientific evidence to help us understand people's lifestyles, and the elements required among the Japanese for keeping healthy.

Among questions surveying their drinking habits, survey participants had to answer the same questions every five years about their frequency of drinking, the types of alcohol they drank, and their intake. Thanks to 140,000 respondents, we've started to see correlations between drinking and the likely development of some diseases.

'For example, let's take diabetes, which is something a lot of drinkers worry about,' says Dr Tsugane. 'If we say that the basic risk for someone who drinks less than once a week is "1", then the risk goes up when the amount drunk exceeds one cup of saké (150g of ethanol) a week.'

Uh-oh . . .

Alcohol consumption and statistical risk of diabetes

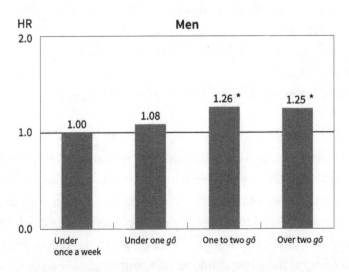

This is the result of a ten-year follow-up study on 15,000 people aged between forty and fifty-nine. For men, the risk of diabetes increased if they exceeded a consumption equivalent of over one gō of saké. For women, on the other hand, the risk was lower. (Waki K, Noda M, Sasaki S, et al., 'Alcohol consumption and other risk factors for self-reported diabetes among middle-aged Japanese: a population-based prospective study in the JPHC study cohort I' in *Diabetic Medicine: A Journal of the British Diabetic Association*, Volume 22, Issue 3, March 2005, 323-331.)

Risks that can be increased or decreased by drinking

Meanwhile, what about Japan's three biggest national killers: heart disease, stroke and cancer?

'If we assign the value 1 to the risk of a non-drinker developing heart disease,' says Dr Tsugane, 'if you drink more, the risk actually drops below 1. On the other hand, when it comes to stroke, the risk goes up if you are consuming more than 300g of ethanol per week. If we look at vascular events as a whole, moderate drinking does not bring higher risks, but actually lowers them a bit.'

I realise you're tempted to start leaping for joy with all the good news, but don't jump the gun. 'Unfortunately, when it comes to the correlation between alcohol intake and all cancers, we know that the more you drink, the higher the risk becomes. International studies of causal correlations have revealed that drinking certainly increases the risk of oral, pharyngeal, laryngeal, oesophageal, colorectal and breast cancer. The Japanese are no exception.'

Treat your liver to a day off

In that case, what should be done in order to keep drinking and stay healthy. Once again, there are some things that the multi-purpose cohort study has made clear. These are that we should stick to a moderate amount of drinking, and maintain a scheme of liver holidays.

You might be getting a sense of déjà vu, but Dr Tsugane's explanation is compelling.

'Looking at the study result, a moderate amount for a Japanese drinker in pure alcohol conversion would be about 20g ethanol a day. That's a 500ml bottle of beer, one *gō* of saké, or two glasses (c.180ml) of wine. You might think "Is that it!?", but considering you can drink up to 150g a week, that's no small amount. Rather than worrying about the total amount per day, you should look at it as a weekly total.'

The liver holiday is also key. Dr Tsugane says that even for those who love nightly drinking sessions more than anything else, a liver holiday is imperative in staying healthy and taking care of your body.

'Even for a small amount, if you drink alcohol every day, the liver will repeatedly break down the alcohol into acetaldehyde.

But routinely processing that "poison" every day is a huge burden on the cells. For men whose pure ethanol intake exceeds 450g per week, those who don't give their liver a day or two off have a mortality risk 1.8 times higher than those who do.[11] You should resolve a drinking plan that allows your liver at least two resting days per week, and do not exceed 150g of ethanol intake. If you are ready to take some risks, then 300g should be the maximum. These are the best measures that we took away from the cohort study.'

If you tell yourself, 'I can't drink tonight, but tomorrow is another day,' a liver holiday shouldn't seem so bad.

B vitamins reduce the risk of disease

Moreover, the study further indicates the possibility that attention to our diet can help lower the risk even further.

'If you eat lots of fruit and vegetables,' says Dr Tsugane, 'that's been reported to lower the risk of, for example, oesophageal cancer (male squamous cell carcinoma). People with a drinking habit may benefit from actively eating these ingredients.'

According to Dr Tsugane, drinkers who have taken a lot of B vitamins, especially vitamin B6, had a lower risk of contracting conditions such as colorectal cancer and myocardial infarction. Foods rich in vitamin B6 include liver and 'red' fish such as tuna and bonito.

'Of course, I don't mean that taking supplements of specific nutrients will bring down the risk of illness. It's important to reduce the salt and carbohydrate intake that can cause lifestyle diseases, and to have a balanced diet. You should also pay attention to the snacks you consume when you are drinking.'

---

11 Marugame, T. et al. 'Patterns of Alcohol Drinking and All-Cause Mortality: Results from a Large-Scale Population-Based Cohort Study in Japan' in *American Journal of Epidemiology* 2007; 165:1039–46.

We also need to bear in mind the importance of regular exercise. The results returned from 140,000 people surveyed shows that those who exercised regularly had a lower risk of developing the three major diseases. Also, those people who exercise routinely drink less or stick to a moderate amount.

Incidentally, it should go without saying that the worst of all combinations with alcohol is smoking. The cohort study indicates that risks of diseases, including cancer, rise dramatically when smokers increase their alcohol intake.

Drink a moderate amount, have liver-resting days, keep to a healthy diet and get some exercise. This is the secret of maintaining a good relationship with alcohol over a long period, while keeping healthy – a conclusion drawn from the data presented by a long-term study of 140,000 people.

Alcohol consumption and statistical risk of cardiovascular disease

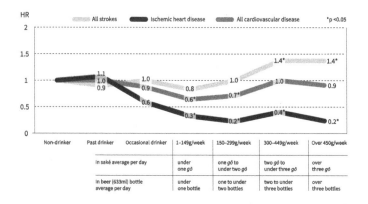

This is the result of a ten-year follow-up study on 19,000 men aged between forty and sixty-nine. If the developing risk of non-drinkers is taken as one, the risk of stroke is high when pure alcohol intake per week is over 300g. In contrast, the risk of ischemic heart disease is low. (Ikehara S, et al. 'Alcohol consumption, social support, and risk of stroke and coronary heart disease among Japanese men: the JPHC Study' in *Alcoholism, Clinical and Experimental Research*, Volume 33, Issue 6, June 2009, 1025-1032.)

Correlation between alcohol intake and overall cancer

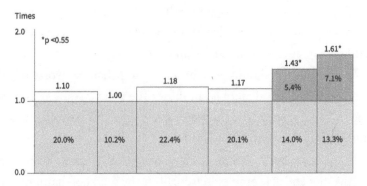

This is the result of a nine- to twelve-year follow-up study on 35,000 men aged between forty and fifty-nine. If the developing risk of occasional drinkers is taken as one, the risk of incidence of cancer increases as the alcohol amount increases. It was also reported that by 'avoiding over two gō of alcohol intake, 12.5 per cent of cancer can be preventable'. (Inoue M, et al., 'Impact of alcohol drinking on total cancer risk: data from a large-scale population-based cohort study in Japan' in *British Journal of Cancer*, Volume 92, Issue 1, 17 January 2005, 182-187.)

'The Best of All Medicines . . . '
up to a point

Expert Adviser: Susumu Higuchi
National Hospital Organisation Kurihama Medical
and Addiction Center

'Saké is the best of all medicines.'

It's a Japanese saying from the olden days, but alcohol is believed to have health benefits if taken in moderation. Indeed, these words have enabled many a drinker to come up with excuses. I am sure many of us have spun that to mean 'it's better to drink than not to drink', even as we reach for a bottle.

And there is data that backs up the idea that moderate drinking can lead to a long life – specialists call it the J-Curve Effect. It's got that name because a chart that shows a horizontal axis of drink intake, and a vertical axis of mortality, will end up looking like the letter J.

That means, that when you drink *moderately*, the mortality rate initially decreases, although once you go over a certain amount, it goes up again. This diagram makes an appearance everywhere to show the beneficial effect of alcohol, so many people, not just the guzzlers, must have seen it.

And I'm one of those guzzlers, gratefully worshipping it as a symbol that brings me reassurance. But if we are going to think about it rationally, how trustworthy is this J-Curve Effect: It is true that the mortality rate decreases, but is that true of all illnesses and all people? What about people with pre-existing conditions, chronic illnesses such as high blood pressure, or those with a stronger tolerance for alcohol than others? There are endless permutations – differences in age, gender, and so on.

I put the question to Susumu Higuchi, the director of the National Hospital Organisation Kurihama Medical and Addiction Center.

The J-Curve Effect does not apply to all illnesses

'Getting straight to the point,' he says, 'the J-Curve Effect can be seen in cohort studies as relevant to the relationship between drinking and all-cause mortality. But it doesn't apply to all illnesses. In other words, there are some illnesses that can be made worse by even a small amount of alcohol. It does not mean that a small amount of alcohol has a beneficial effect on everything.'

A cohort study, as we've seen before, is a long-term epidemiological study of a group of the general public. According to Dr Higuchi, studies of drinking and healthy risks in both Japan and the West have found a 'J-Curve' correlation between alcohol intake and all-cause mortality. 'A report published in 1996,' he notes, 'analysed fourteen studies of people in the West, and showed that the mortality rate of those with an average daily alcohol intake of 19g was lower than that of non-alcohol drinkers, in both genders.' [12]

---

12 Holman, C.D. et al. 'Meta-analysis of alcohol and all-cause mortality: a validation of NHMRC recommendations' in the *Medical Journal of Australia*, 1996; 164: 141–145.

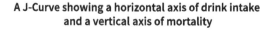

A J-Curve showing a horizontal axis of drink intake and a vertical axis of mortality

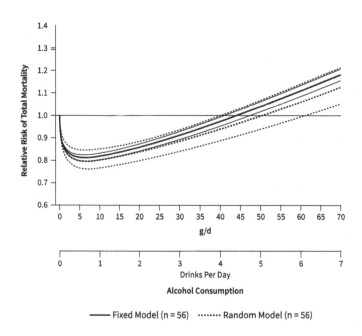

A similar large-scale cohort study in Japan also showed that moderate drinking decreased the risks of mortality.[13] It was a follow-up to a study of approximately 110,000 men and women between the ages of forty and seventy-nine, and found that the all-cause mortality of those with an average daily alcohol intake of less than 23g (less than one cup of saké), have the lowest risks.

Such reports from both Japan and overseas have led to the popular belief that moderate drinking can reduce the mortality rate. 'It's true,' adds Dr Higuchi, 'that these cohort studies show a low mortality rate for those who drink a little bit, but there is no

13 Lin, Y. et al. 'Alcohol consumption and mortality among middle-aged and elderly Japanese men and women' in *Annals of Epidemiology* 2005; 15: 590–597.

indication of a causal relationship with drinking. Furthermore, we only see this J-Curve Effect in middle-aged men and women in developed countries.'

Even a small amount of drinking can be a risk for high blood pressure and dyslipidaemia

So Dr Higuchi has revealed that the J-Curve Effect is only seen with certain illnesses. All this time, I have believed that saké was 'the best of all medicines' and that 'moderate drinking is good for you', but now he's got me worried. So, what risks for which diseases does even a small amount of alcohol carry?

'The kind of illnesses that can be exacerbated even by a small amount of alcohol include, in the main, high blood pressure, dyslipidaemia, cerebral haemorrhage, and breast cancer (in the over-forties). In the graphs for these diseases, the risk rises steadily in step with the alcohol intake. In other words, even a small amount of alcohol increases the risk. Breast cancer has a strong genetic component, but even so, drinking increases its occurrence compared with the rate of occurrence for non-drinkers.

'As for cirrhosis of the liver, the graphs show an exponential trend. The more you drink, for sure, the more the risk goes up, but whereas there's a small increase with a small amount, once you cross a certain threshold, the risk shoots up.'

Dr Higuchi's litany of illnesses was frightening to hear. High blood pressure, dyslipidaemia and breast cancer are familiar terms for those over middle age. But in that case, why is there still a belief that moderate drinking *decreases* the risks in all-cause mortality?

Correlation between alcohol intake and mortality risk (Japanese)

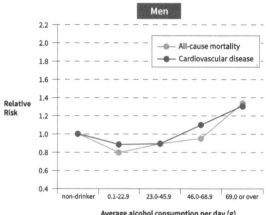

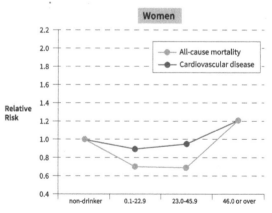

According to cohort studies in Japan, the mortality rates of all-cause and cardiovascular disease were confirmed to have a tendency to be lowered by moderate alcohol consumption. (Lin, Y., Kikuchi S., Tamakoshi A. et al., 'Alcohol consumption and mortality among middle-aged and elderly Japanese men and women' in *Annals of Epidemiology*, Volume 15, Issue 8, September 2005, 590-597.)

'As you can see in the graph (below), the disease rates for ischemic heart disease, including heart attacks and angina, strokes and type-2 diabetes, all decrease with a slight amount of drinking. Heart attacks, in particular, have a significantly large effect on overall mortality rates. It's because of the decrease in that particular risk that the general risk is reduced, as heart attacks have a bigger impact on mortality than some of the other problems I mentioned earlier. That's what creates the J-Curve Effect.'

Dr Higuchi adds that there is also a lower risk for cognitive function decline in the elderly. Okay, then – so how should we actually interpret these results, and what effect should it have on our drinking?

'It's certainly true,' he says, 'that you should limit your alcohol intake if you have a chronic disease like high blood pressure, dyslipidaemia, or poor liver function, or if you have relatives with breast cancer. The risks for such people increase even with a small amount of alcohol. Even so, drinking has a social function, and a pleasurable release from daily stress. It's also true that people with, say, high blood pressure should limit their intake of alcohol, but there is no need to be over-sensitive about it.'

So watch out, but don't be too oversensitive. That's good to hear. As long as we do not overindulge and keep to small amounts, alcohol is nothing to be afraid of.

Patterns of correlation between alcohol intake and risks

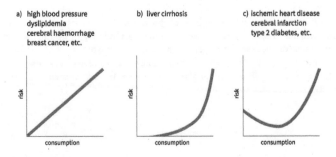

a) high blood pressure
dyslipidemia
cerebral haemorrhage
breast cancer, etc.

b) liver cirrhosis

c) ischemic heart disease
cerebral infarction
type 2 diabetes, etc.

Blush response – watch out if you get red-faced

So far, Dr Higuchi's explanations have made it clear that the risks from drinking are contingent on pre-existing conditions. But what about people without a high level of alcohol tolerance, who get red-faced soon after they start drinking?

'If your face turns red after drinking alcohol,' he replies, 'which is to say, if you have a naturally low ability to metabolise alcohol, you need to be careful. We know that people with such a condition have a higher risk of drinking-related illnesses like oesophageal cancer. They should pursue a relatively limited alcohol intake.'

Dr Higuchi adds that the elderly carry even higher risks.

'Older people have slower rates of metabolising alcohol and they hold less water in their body, so their blood alcohol concentration can get high. A lot of them also have chronic illnesses. The risk of falling over when drunk is also higher. There are quite a few cases in which they end up with broken bones, leaving them bed-ridden in turn.'

So drinking for the elderly is fraught with dangers. I am yet to be categorised as 'old', but it's true that the older I get, the longer it takes me to sober up. Dr Higuchi's words hit me hard, and I asked him if ultimately it was better not to drink at all?

Dr Higuchi waves off my pessimistic response.

'There's no need to force yourself to stop drinking altogether,' he says. Instead, he advises those who drink to excess to start by reducing the amount.

'I could tell patients at the hospital with alcohol-related ill-health to just stop,' he continues, 'but if drinking has become a habit, then completely stopping would just make them more stressed. A command to cease all alcohol consumption can actually have the opposite effect. What should they do? They should reduce their intake within reason. It's important that the person should decide themselves what kind of amount that means.'

Reduce your intake even a little bit! Keep a record!

'We often hear that the recommended guidelines for alcohol intake is about 20g pure alcohol a day (one 500ml bottle of beer or one cup of saké) for men, but it's hard to cut down your usual amount to that if you're drinking three times as much a day. Therefore, the important thing to do is to set a target and reduce the amount, even a little bit. Reducing your alcohol intake, even a little, will reduce the risk.

'So set a small target. If you're drinking two cups a day of saké, make it one and a half. The important thing is that you give yourself a star in your notebook for clearing your target. That will lead you to naturally keep track of your intake. Small daily successes will help reduce the amount you drink naturally.'

It sounds like a diet, but keeping a record works for drinking, too, and increases the success rate for reducing consumption. 'Telling everybody about it can also be effective,' suggests Dr Higuchi. 'Once you've made a declaration, you are more likely to be held to it.'

I see – I may not be able to give up drinking altogether, but I can still do this.

As he mentions, the guideline for daily alcohol intake is 20g in pure alcohol conversion *for men*, but for women it is just 10g – one small beer can. You're probably thinking: is that it!? It is hard for the habitual drinker to drop down to such a small amount, but if you are aware that you are drinking too much, it's worth knowing what amount is actually considered reasonable.

However, when we start reducing our drinking and coming up with 'liver holidays', we can develop the tendency for compensation drinking, making excuses like: 'I didn't drink at all yesterday, so it's okay to drink twice as much today.'

'If you compare drinking a moderate amount of 20g a day for a week,' says Dr Higuchi, 'and drinking 140g all in one binge, the latter is by far the most taxing on the body. It is important to have liver holidays, but also to keep to a daily moderate amount, rather than drinking a week's worth in one night.'

Dr Higuchi thinks that the idea of a liver holiday (*kyūkanbi*) is a uniquely Japanese term.

'In Western countries,' he says, 'they have the idea of non-drinking days, but to avoid alcohol dependency rather than giving the liver a rest.'

So keep steady, keep to a moderate amount every day, and if you drink too much, try to reduce the amount, even by a little. After all, there cannot be a wiser way than this to reduce the risk of various diseases. But now that we know the statistics behind the J-Curve Effect, we must bear in mind that even no amount of alcohol, be it 'moderate' or even less, can ever be entirely safe.

'Saké is the best of all medicines' comes with a lot of small print.

Flushed Away – do you get a red face?

Expert Adviser: Yōichi Kakibuchi
Tokyo Alcoholic Medical Treatment Synthesis Center,
Narimasu Welfare Hospital

There are two kinds of people in the world: Those who get a red face after drinking and those who don't.

I get envious of a woman whose face gets flushed after half a glass of beer, turning the colour of cherry blossoms. It's such a sexy look!

I might get flushed like that several times a year, but it takes twice as much alcohol to do that to me as it does the average person.

If you do get red-faced and cry off drinking, people are more readily convinced, and stop trying to top up your glass. But because my complexion stays the same, people can assume that I can drink more, and even when I am reaching the maximum, I find my glass keeps refilling itself. That leads me to drink too much every single time.[14]

So what's the difference between those who get red-faced and those who don't? Based on my experience, among those who can

---

14 Translators' note – in Japan it's customary to fill others' glasses, rather than your own, which can make it easier for drinkers in company to enable each other.

handle their drink, there are a lot fewer people who get red-faced. But there are some drinkers who do get a flushed face, so it may be that there is not necessarily a correlation between the amount you can drink and the degree to which you go red.

I wonder if getting a red face is some sort of physiological signal, and put the question to Yōichi Kakibuchi from the Tokyo Alcoholic Medical Treatment Synthesis Center, Narimasu Welfare Hospital.

It's all about the acetaldehyde!

'The combination of all these symptoms,' says Dr Kakibuchi, 'including facial flushing, rising blood pressure, cold sweats and palpitations, is called Alcohol Flushing. The major cause of a red face is the toxic effect of acetaldehyde, a substance created when the body metabolises alcohol. The acetaldehyde causes the blood capillaries to expand, turning the face red. It strongly stimulates the sympathetic nerve, which increases the heart rate, and that in turn can lead to a rise in blood pressure, cold sweats and muscle tension. Additionally, alcohol increases the blood flow, which can also help make the face appear flushed.'

So we're back to the blasted acetaldehyde, the same stuff that causes hangovers. And a long-term skin condition with a red nose and cheeks, caused by chronic Alcohol Flushing, is known medically as rosacea, although in Japanese we call it *sakéyake*, the 'alcohol burn'.

But everybody's body creates acetaldehyde when they drink, so why do only some of us get red-faced?

'Actually,' he says, 'the difference between those who go red and those who don't is hugely affected by aldehyde dehydrogenases (ALDH), the substances that break down acetaldehyde. One of them, ALDH2, has an activity dependent on genetic factors

– the strength of your ALDH2 is determined at birth, into one of three types.'

Aldehyde dehydrogenase activity is the key

It turns out that 90 per cent of the alcohol you ingest is metabolised in your liver. There, the alcohol (ethanol) is broken down into acetaldehyde by alcohol dehydrogenases. Then, the aldehyde dehydrogenases (ALDH, in three types 1, 2, and 3) convert the acetaldehyde into a non-toxic acetic acid, which is discharged from the liver (see page 57). Among the ALDHs, ALDH1 and ALDH2 don't differ much between people, but ALDH2 is the key to determining if a person can drink a lot or not.

Let's find out the differences between the three types of ALDH2 activities.

Normal ALDH2 (NN) has stable and normal ALDH2 activities. It is inherited from both parents' type N, regarded to have a high ability to break down alcohol. These people are known to be guzzlers and they themselves admit it. Most of them don't get red faces when they get drunk.

Normal and Inactive ALDH2 (ND, also called Low-Active), is the second type. If you have this, you have inherited 'N' with a high breakdown ability, and 'D' with a low-active ability. Such people can drink, but they can get drunk easily. If they are not exposed to alcohol on a regular basis, they can get red-faced if they touch the stuff.

The final type is the Inactive ALDH (DD), which is where you inherit the inactive type D from both parents. It would be fairer to say that they can't drink, rather than that they get drunk easily. Most of them will get red-faced, and they can get that way even by just easting *narazuke* – vegetables pickled in saké.

In East Asia, approximately 50 per cent of Mongoloid races like the Japanese have the Active type, 40 per cent have the Low-Active, and 10 per cent Inactive. Conversely, almost 100 per cent of white people and black people have the Active type.

'There are anti-alcohol drugs,' says Dr Kakibuchi, 'that block the activity of ASDH2 in everybody. In other words, we can medically induce the Inactive state. Then, even if someone is genetically Active, even a small amount of alcohol will give them palpitations and a red face as if they are Inactive. Sometimes we have alcoholic patients who sneak out of the hospital to get a drink at a convenience store or somewhere like that, but because they turn red so quickly, we immediately know that they have snuck in a drink. Actually, they don't just turn red, but they get heavy symptoms, like headaches, nausea and giddiness.'

Hmm . . . I think I'd like to avoid those drugs . . .

Three ALDH2 Active types and alcohol tolerance

Active type	Alcohol tolerance and facial flushing	Incidence		
		White	Black	Mongoloid (Japanese)
Normal (NN type)	Strong alcohol tolerance Non-flushing	100%	100%	c.50%
Low Active (ND type)	Slight alcohol tolerance Tendency to flush	0%	0%	c.40%
Inactive (DD type)	Weak alcohol tolerance Flushing	0%	0%	c.10%

As everyone has different facial reactions, be careful!

As you can see from these cases, there is a strong correlation between facial flushing and ALDH2 activity. However, as I mentioned earlier, there do seem to be cases where a person's resistance to alcohol (≠ALDH2 activity) and facial flushing do not match. Why is that?

'Like I said, acetaldehyde is the *main cause* of facial flushing,' explains Dr Kakibuchi. 'So those people with active ALDH2 are mainly okay, and those with inactive ALDH2 get red-faced. But reaction in the blood capillaries varies from person to person, and in some cases, they don't match up. It is rare, but there are some cases of inactive-type people not getting facial flushing.'

Low-active types are susceptible to oesophageal cancer

Now I sort of get the correlation between ALDH2 and facial flushing. So is there anything in particular that people of each type should be aware of?

'Active-type people are strong drinkers,' replies Dr Kakibuchi, 'and so they can easily slip into habitual heavy drinking and turn into alcoholics. Inactive types can swiftly fall into a critical condition, so do not ever force them to drink. If you are one of them, you should firmly decline the offer of alcoholic drinks, even amid the peer pressure of a drinking party. And as I said, not all Inactive-type people will have tell-tale red faces – if you force them to drink just because they don't have a red face, they may suffer acute alcohol poisoning. Please be careful.'

The biggest problem, however, comes from the Low-Active types.

'They're the ones you need to be most careful of,' says Dr Kakibuchi. 'If they are low-active and can drink a reasonable amount, they are textbook cases of the people who think you can train yourself to take more drink. They have lower ALDH2 activity by nature, and aren't strong drinkers, but if they repeatedly metabolise alcohol, their ALDH2 activity will improve. In other words, they can increase their alcohol tolerance by drinking more.'

But here's the problem. Alcohol is basically broken down by ALDH2; when you drink a large amount you also induce drug metabolising enzymes, which contribute to the processing of alcohol by the body.

'Even for the low-active type,' says Dr Kakibuchi, 'routine drinking will encourage enzyme induction, which increases the ability to break alcohol down and decreases the amount of facial flushing.' Hearing that, you'd be forgiven for thinking it was good news and that you can drink more, but it's not that simple.

'Originally, people with low-active type ALDH2 have a low alcohol tolerance,' continues Dr Kakibuchi. 'Even if your alcohol tolerance increases through enzyme induction, you still have more alcohol left behind than someone with an active type ALDH2, and so there is a risk of a longer physical exposure to toxic acetaldehyde. As a result, you have a higher risk of pharyngeal or oesophageal cancer. In fact, when patients are admitted to the hospital I work at [a dedicated alcohol facility], there is a high chance that we find diseases like oesophageal cancer during their stay.'

In addition, a cohort study by the National Cancer Center Japan showed a strong correlation between drinking and oesophageal cancer. Compared to those who do not drink at all, those who drink a couple of cups of saké a day are 2.6 times more likely to get the cancer, and those who drink more, 4.6 times more at risk.

The same study also investigated the correlation between physical traits and facial flushing. The results showed that if a heavy smoker who gets facial flushes when drinking increases their alcohol intake, they also increase their risk of oesophageal cancer.

Drinking and the risk of oesophageal cancer by the degree of smoking and reaction to alcohol

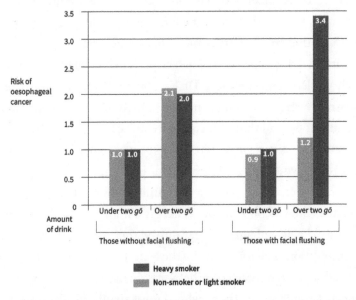

Heavy smokers who tend to get facial flushing have higher risk of oesophageal cancer with higher alcohol intake. (Source: National Cancer Center Japan cohort study. Ishiguro S, Sasazuki S, Inoue M, et al., 'Effect of alcohol consumption, cigarette smoking and flushing response on oesophageal cancer risk: a population-based cohort study (JPHC study)' *Cancer Letters*, Volume 275, Issue 2, 18 March 2009, 240-246.)

Find out your type through genetic testing

If you're an inactive type, you're best off not touching alcohol at all, but those with low-active type ALDH2 who have become inured to heavier drinking through enzyme induction need to take care. But how do you know if you are a low-active type?

'The best way to find out is through genetic screening,' says Dr Kakibuchi. 'There is a large possibility that you may think you are an active type but turn out to be low-active. To avoid the risk of cancer, I recommend you should get a check-up at a specialist organisation as an initial investment. These days, all this information is available as part of a general genetic screening.'

I can well imagine that there are many people with East Asian ethnic backgrounds who believe that they have active-type ALDH2, even if they are actually low-active, particularly if they have a long history of drinking. It would be worthwhile for such people to get their genes checked as a personal investment in their health, as Dr Kakibuchi suggests.

If a full-scale genetic screening is beyond your budget, you can try an alcohol patch test. It's very easy – saturate some cotton wool with medical alcohol, fix it to the inner side of your upper arm with tape for seven minutes, and then check the colour of your skin, both as soon as you take it off, and again ten minutes later. If the skin is red when you take it off, you are inactive. If it has turned red after ten minutes, you are a low-active type.

But even then, since there are a few low-active types as mentioned above, who don't turn red, if you want a truly accurate diagnosis, the genetic screening is the way to go.

'Either way,' says Dr Kakibuchi, 'knowing your ALDH2 type will be an opportunity to avoid some alcohol-related illnesses and to consider the way that you drink. Please give it some thought.'

There must be many drinkers who became heavy drinkers after heady youthful days of big parties and beer-chugging. But we would all like to avoid a situation where you mistakenly believe you are a robust drinker, only to discover that you are facing a higher risk of contracting cancer. On the other hand, some of you might have found yourself in a situation where your boss forces you to have another one, on the grounds that you haven't turned red yet. You can avoid such situations if you know your ALDH2 type. It's crucial to understand what your type is, in order to enjoy drinking healthily.

Yellow Peril – how turmeric can cause liver damage

Expert Adviser: Shinichi Asabe
Jichi Medical University Saitama Medical Center

There are a lot of hard-core drinkers who swear by taking a vitamin supplement or a health drink containing turmeric. I can safely say that I've heard this described as common sense and a 'pre-drink ritual'.

I've found myself that if I take a turmeric drink before alcohol, I don't get drunk so quickly, and wake up feeling much better the morning after. So I am a convert to the power of turmeric.

However, in early 2017, a piece went viral on the internet suggesting that turmeric, the big cure-all for the ill effects of alcohol, had no such power. It caused an uproar, not least because it wasn't a vague rumour, but a peer-reviewed article from the *Journal of Medicinal Chemistry*, a respected academic publication from the USA.[15] The paper didn't deny the beneficial effect of curcumin, the active ingredient in turmeric, however, so news articles provided a bit more context, and the excitement died down.

---

15 Nelson, K.M. et al. 'The Essential Medicinal Chemistry of Curcumin' in *Journal of Medicinal Chemistry* 2017; 60: 1620–1637.

But then I heard that the turmeric wonder-herb should indeed be avoided if you have a liver function problem. There is a possibility that it might have an adverse effect on people with fatty livers. One in three Japanese adults are said to suffer from this problem (see page 48) so this is not somebody else's problem.

Turmeric is something that drinkers have come to rely on, but should we avoid taking it . . . ? I put the question to Shinichi Asabe from Jichi Medical University Saitama Medical Center.

Turmeric reported as a cause of liver disorder

'There are two reasons why I wouldn't recommend turmeric to those with liver function problems,' says Dr Asabe. 'One is that there are reports that turmeric does cause liver disorder. There's been a lot more on this about turmeric than there has about many other health foods and traditional medicines.

'A few years ago, the Japan Society of Hepatology conducted research about drug-induced liver damage caused by something other than medicine administered at hospitals – meaning traditional medicine and health foods. The results showed a variety of causes, but the biggest cause turned out to be turmeric. Turmeric was responsible for 24.8 per cent of drug-induced liver damage, by far the largest factor. [16] Ever since, the idea that you need to take care with turmeric has been gaining ground.

'The research included reports of three fatal cases. One of them was a patient with acute hepatitis, which had been caused by turmeric. It led to multiple organ failure, and then death.'

Incidentally, according to the Japan Society of Hepatology, of those who developed drug-induced hepatitis, 91 per cent were habitual

16 Onji, M. et al. 'Investigation of drug-induced hepatopathy by folk medicine and by health food' in *Kanzo* 2005; 46(3): 142–148.

users of traditional medicine and health food, often daily. It took, on average, 160 days of usage before the disease manifested itself, but in 23.6 per cent of the cases, the disease developed within a month.

Drinking boiled-down turmeric root landed a patient in hospital

It gets worse. According to a paper on the characteristics of health hazards and patient backgrounds related to traditional medicines and health supplements, published in 2013, turmeric was ranked as the number-three cause of adverse drug reactions to any individual health-food ingredient. [17]

Drinkers have made a terrible mistake. We've been drinking turmeric in the belief it will heighten liver function, but it turns out to be one of the causes of drug-induced liver damage.

Dr Asabe has even had patients who are living proof.

Folk remedies and health foods that cause liver disorder

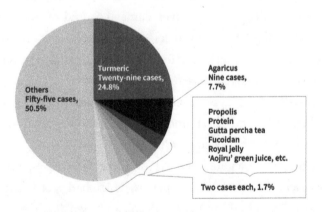

Of 117 cases and sixty-nine kinds of medicinal substances, turmeric was involved in twenty-nine cases, nearly a quarter. (Morikazu Onji, et al., 'Investigation of drug-induced hepatopathy by folk medicine and by health food' in *Kanzo*, Volume 46, Issue 3, 2005, 142-148.)

---

17 Koike, M. et al. 'Kenkō supplement ni yoru kenkō higai no genjō to kanja haikei no tokuchō' in *Japanese Journal of Drug Information* 2013; 14(4): 134–143.

'At Jichi Medical University Saitama Medical Center, where I work, we have had many patients with illnesses that other hospitals could not find the cause of. When I get a patient with liver dysfunction and hugely abnormal liver function values, including gamma-GTP, I would consider the possibility of drug-induced liver damage. In fact, when I get patients like that, I always ask the following three questions. "Are you taking any prescription drugs? Do you take any supplements or herbal medicines? And do you drink turmeric?"

'In fact, we had an outpatient the other day, in his fifties, who had taken so much turmeric that he had developed liver damage. Since he stopped taking it, the values have improved.

'His liver function had deteriorated so much that he had to stay in the hospital. But he hadn't been taking just a supplement with turmeric in it. He had chosen a really hard-core method – he bought turmeric root on the internet, boiled it down and drank it. When I heard that, I realised he was ingesting a huge amount of turmeric, and I asked him to stop. The values improved, and he left the hospital.'

So do all of us need to worry about drug-induced liver damage, caused by turmeric?

'We know that people with some sort of pre-existing liver problems tend to get drug-induced liver damage. So those are the people who need to watch out, like people with fatty liver and habitual drinkers of alcohol. I would not recommend turmeric to those people.'

Is the iron content also bad for your liver?

Dr Asabe would also recommend that people with fatty livers avoid turmeric because of its iron content.

'There are some turmeric supplements that contain relatively large amounts of iron,' he says. 'Iron is known to have an adverse effect on someone who has liver problems, such as hepatitis C and fatty liver. Iron is known to be effective for anaemia, but with excessive intake it ends up getting stored in the liver, which then generates active oxygen, damages the liver cells and aggravates the inflammation. Fibrosis (see page 49) can harden the liver, which makes the possibility of cirrhosis and liver cancer more likely. From my experience of treating patients, most of the people with fatty liver have an excessive amount of iron in their blood. Therefore, those with a fatty liver would be better off watching their turmeric intake. The same goes for basket clams (*corbicula*), which also contain a lot of iron.

'Many people believe that they should take in a lot of iron, but that only really applies to women. Women might need an iron supplement if they are menstruating, but men rarely experience an iron deficiency. In fact, people who routinely consume alcohol and have fatty livers tend to have excess iron in their blood stream, so they need to be careful.'

There must be quite a few people who make a habit of taking turmeric and corbicula supplements, believing they will heighten liver function. Some might even eat liver as a food because it's 'iron-rich', but that might not be good for their own liver at all. That comes as quite a shock . . .

Don't worry too much, but . . .

So now I want to know if we'd be better off not drinking turmeric at all.

'If you're the kind of person, without liver dysfunction,' says Dr Asabe, 'who occasionally gets one of those turmeric shots from a convenience store, then you don't need to worry about it too much. In fact, there are some reports that confirm that if you ingest curcumin, which is contained in turmeric, thirty minutes before drinking alcohol, you can suppress the rise of blood acetaldehyde levels. [18] So, certainly, many people feel it's effective.'

The reason why there are so many reports about turmeric causing drug-induced liver damage is presumably because there are so many people who drink turmeric. However, you need to avoid taking highly concentrated doses, such as you would find in 'decocted juice' – an extract of turmeric made by boiling down the roots. Nor should you take refined turmeric powder for a long period of time. There are a few incidences where a health food can cause problems after a single dose, but most of the time, it's continuous ingestion that damages the liver. Also, anyone with liver problems, such as fatty liver, should avoid it.

'That applies to any health food, not just turmeric,' says Dr Asabe, 'but there is hardly anything that doesn't have some kind of side effect. If you are worried about your health, I recommend you consult with your doctor before taking health supplements, and if you continue to take them, make sure you have a regular check-up.'

Even with health foods, it's risky to rely on your own judgement. These days, you can buy some medicines on the internet, and supplements at a convenience store. It makes it easier to jump onto what is believed to be 'effective', but we should never forget there are dangers in assuming that everything will be beneficial.

So let's think again about how we live with turmeric.

18 Sasaki, H. 'Innovative preparation of curcumin for improved oral bioavailability' in *Biological & Pharmaceutical Bulletin* 2011; 34(5): 660–665.

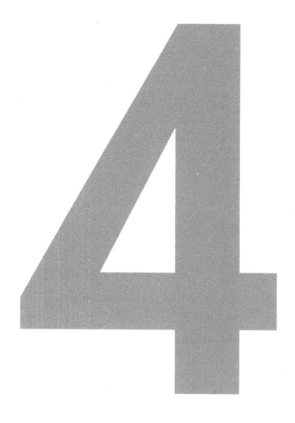

FAQs & Figures – the whys and hows of drinking

Fill Her Up – how can you drink so much beer but not water?

Expert Adviser: Masashi Matsushima
Tōkai University School of Medicine

When the thermometer is hitting 35°C at the height of summer, the drinkers declare, 'In weather like this, we need beer! Beer!'

Even when we're sweating profusely, a gulp of ice-cold beer can make us feel like the body-core is being cooled. Beer is the best in summer. It's so tasty that I can find I've downed three large glasses before I know it.

I look at the line of empty pint glasses in front of me, and I wonder, how can I drink so much beer, but not the same amount of water?

I am only 152cm tall. How can I stack three 700ml glasses, 2.1 litres, of beer inside such a little body? On the other hand, if I try to drink water, my storage capacity is dramatically less – maybe one 300ml glass. I ask male friends, and they say a litre at most is the best they can manage.

Because it puzzled me for a while, I looked it up online, and found a bunch of other people asking the same question. Some answers suggested that we can drink more alcohol because it's absorbed in the stomach, but is that true?

To unravel the mystery that has stumped many a drinker, I put the question to Masashi Matsushima of Tōkai University School of Medicine, who has an expert knowledge of the mechanism of the digestive system, including the stomach and the intestines.

Alcohol absorbed in the stomach is c.5%

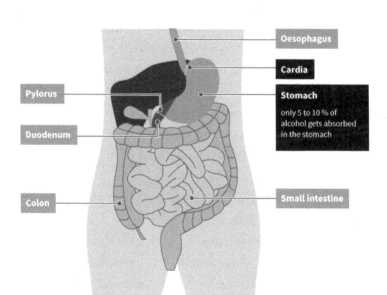

Alcohol can be absorbed through the stomach, but only 5 to 10 per cent of it. The rest is absorbed in the small intestine.

Only a small amount of alcohol is absorbed through the stomach

To start with, is it really true that we can't drink much water but can drink a lot more beer?

'I've never measured how much beer people can drink,' says Professor Matsushima, 'but some people, just like you, can drink three or four large glasses. On the other hand, there was a water load test that investigated how much water people can drink. The result showed that the amount of water a person can drink in a single session is 1 to 1.5 litres at most.[19] Of course, it varies from person to person, but it seems to be true that some people can drink more beer than water.'

So why can we drink more beer?

'It's true, to an extent, that alcohol is absorbed in the stomach. But the alcohol absorbed in the stomach only accounts for 5 to 10 per cent at most, and the rest is absorbed by the small intestine. So the effect is limited. For starters, beer is largely made of water, which cannot be absorbed in the stomach, so it mostly stays in the stomach. Therefore, this internet theory that you saw, that you can drink more alcohol because it is absorbed in the stomach, cannot be the main factor.'

So, although there is an element of truth in the internet rumour, it's only a supplemental factor.

'In fact, the alcohol suppresses the excretory function of the stomach, making it harder for it to process everything out. Research carried out by the University of Zurich in Switzerland, as well as in some other institutions, has shown that the higher the alcohol content, the greater the suppression of the stomach's excretory function.[20] This is believed to happen through the receptor cholecystokinin (CCK), a kind of digestive hormone.'

What!? I cannot let go of this information! Beer's alcohol by volume (ABV) is only 5 per cent or so, but it can still suppress the

---

19 Jones et al. 'The water load test: observations from healthy controls and patients with functional dyspepsia' in the *American Journal of Physiology. Gastrointestinal and Liver Physiology*; 2003: 284, G896–G904.

20 Heinrich, H. et al. 'Effect on gastric function and symptoms of drinking wine, black tea or schnapps with a Swiss cheese fondue: randomised control crossover trial' in the *British Medical Journal*; 2010: 341, c6731.

excretory function of the stomach. Hmm, this should mean that we would be able to drink even less of it, not more. So what is causing the phenomenon of being able to drink more?

'Gastrin' enhances the excretory function of the stomach

'There has yet to be a clear theory,' says Professor Matsushima, 'but the existence of a hormone called gastrin, secreted by the stomach, may have something to do with it.

'G cells, found in the pyloric glands around the antrum (the exit from the stomach), secrete a hormone called gastrin. The main functions of gastrin are to increase the muscle motility of the stomach, to stimulate the secretion of gastric acid, to stimulate the secretion of pepsinogen, gastric wall cell proliferation, and to stimulate the secretion of insulin. In addition, gastrin is reported to suppress the movement near the entrance of the stomach, and stimulate movement near the exit. [21] This allows the stomach to hold a large amount of contents, and helps discharge contents near the outlet.

'According to research by the University of Essen in Germany, along with some other institutions, beer can have the effect of stimulating the secretion of gastrin.[22] It is possible that drinking beer heightens the excretory function of the stomach. As a result, you can drink more.

'The researchers found that this effect could be seen with brewed liquors, including beer and wine, which use yeast to convert sugar into alcohol, although beer seemed to be the most powerful. We can't confirm that there is a similar effect from

---

21 Thomas, P. et al. 'Hormonal control of gastrointestinal motility' in *World Journal of Surgery*; 1979: 3, 545–552.

22 Singer, M. et al. 'Action of beer and its ingredients on gastric acid secretion and release of gastrin in humans' in *Gastroenterology*; 1991: 101, 935–942.

distilled spirits or watered-down alcohol. But we don't know what the actual ingredient is that helps the secretion of gastrin. It is believed that there is some sort of volatile component that comes out of the brewing process. [23] So there is a chance that gastrin is the factor that makes us able to drink more beer. Some other reports have said that other ingredients found in beer, such as aperidine, directly stimulate gastrointestinal motility.' [24]

It seems that gastrin certainly has some effect, but the precise details are yet to be unravelled. We shall have to await future research.

Carbonic acid helps alcohol absorption

According to Professor Matsushima, the carbonic acid in beer also helps alcohol absorption.

'Drinks that contain carbonic acid have better alcohol absorption,' he said. 'The University of Manchester in the UK compared straight vodka, vodka mixed with water and vodka mixed with fizzy water. The result showed that subjects who tried the third variety – vodka with *carbonated* water – had the highest levels of blood alcohol concentration.[25] A carbonated drink with a low alcohol content still has a higher alcohol absorption.

'This suggests that beer, a carbonated low-ABV drink, has a higher level of alcohol absorption than other alcoholic drinks. Having said that, beer's alcohol content is still only 5 per cent, so

23 Teyssen, S. et al. 'Maleic acid and succinic acid in fermented alcoholic beverages are the stimulants of gastric acid secretion' in the *Journal of Clinical Investigation*, 1999: 103, 707–713.

24 Nahoko, Y. et al. 'Structural Determination of Two Active Compounds That Bind to the Muscarinic M3 Receptor in Beer' in *Alcoholism, Clinical and Experimental Research* 2007: 31, 9S–14S.

25 Robert, C., and Robinson, S.P. 'Alcohol Concentration and Carbonation of Drinks: the Effect on Blood Alcohol levels' in *Journal of Forensic and Legal Medicine*, 2007: 14, 398–405.

that doesn't account for the body's ability to absorb the other 95 per cent. So it's hard to say that this would be the main factor.'

Incidentally, Professor Matsushima says that the succinic and maleic acids contained in beer can stimulate the secretion of gastric acid. If you go to a Japanese inn, you might find yourself served with plum wine (*umeshu*) or Japanese plum wine (*sumomoshu*) as a dinnertime aperitif. Both contain large amounts of succinic acid and maleic acid, which help the secretion of gastric acid and the motility of the stomach. It turns out that drinking beer at the start of a party isn't just about its refreshing and smooth quality.

Now we know that gastrin may be responsible for our ability to drink more beer. Having said that, if you drink glass after glass just because you can drink beer more easily, you will surely end up with a hangover. That's because beer also has a diuretic effect – it makes you pee more. Professor Matsushima, back in his student days, used to get through 20 litres of beer in a session with his three friends, so he has first-hand experience.

'You will suffer the next day after drinking too much beer,' he says, smiling wryly. 'You need to hydrate to spare yourself from a horrible morning after.' But because beer mostly comprises water, drinking beer with a water chaser is difficult. At the very least, we shouldn't forget to have some water at the end of the night out, or after we get home.

Shakes on a Plane – is in-flight drinking dangerous?

Expert Adviser: Hirofumi Ōkoshi
Travel Medicine Center, Nishi Shinbashi Clinic

Do you ever think you get drunker faster when you fly? Not only regular drinkers, but occasional drinkers can feel that they get plastered on a plane. I once got tipsy and red-faced, even though that hardly ever happens, on just one tin of beer when I was flying. It was a big deal for me, a hooch hound who usually has beer as a chaser for the hard stuff. Ever since, I have stayed away from alcohol on planes.

But why do we get drunk faster in the air than on the ground? It can't just be the giddy feeling of going on holiday . . . But if you look up the facts about drinking on a plane, you swiftly discover people pointing out there might a correlation with the so-called economy-class syndrome. Getting drunk easily is one thing, but it's no laughing matter if it's also a matter of life and death.

I put the question to Hirofumi Ōkoshi from the Travel Medical Center, Nishi Shinbashi Clinic.

'I advise you not to drink'

'I think many people on planes feel like drinking alcohol,' says

Dr Ōkoshi, 'probably helped by the feeling of liberation when travelling. But I advise you not to drink.'

What? He just shut us down from drinking altogether, and in such a soft tone. Is it really that dangerous to drink on an aeroplane that it requires a medical ban?

'When a plane takes off, it flies at a cruising altitude of about 10,000 metres. During the flight, it draws in air from the outside, and controls the pressure with a pressurisation device. The air pressure inside the plane is about 0.8 atmospheres (atm), coming down to about 0.74atm, which is equivalent to the air pressure you would experience at the fifth station of Mount Fuji (about 2000 to 2500 metres above sea level). If the air pressure gets any lower than that, the incidences of altitude sickness start to go up, so they try to make sure it doesn't drop any further.

'But when we lower the air pressure, the partial pressure of the oxygen is reduced. Specifically, the partial pressure of the oxygen in the cabin is reduced to about 80 per cent of what it would be on the ground. To put it simply, the amount of oxygen you breathe in is reduced by 20 per cent when you are flying, compared to when you are on the ground. In such an environment, the body tries to cope by breathing more and raising the pulse, but still, the blood oxygen concentration (oxygen saturated concentration) drops to about 92 to 93 per cent – a state of hypoxemia. If oxygen saturated concentration drops to 90 per cent, that's a hypoxemia danger level. In other words, you are already on the redline. This low oxygen level is one of the reasons why you feel you get drunk quicker than usual.'

Low oxygen, high drunkenness

There are some pundits who claim that the reason you get drunk quickly on an aeroplane is because of the low air pressure in the cabin. The peripheral blood vessels dilate, the blood circulates more quickly, and that contributes to the drunkenness. Moreover, they say that the low oxygen conditions mean that the oxygen required to metabolise alcohol is in shorter supply, slowing down the processing of alcohol. But Dr Ōkoshi says that there has not yet been any medical evidence to back up these theories.

But what *is* happening to our bodies in a low oxygen environment?

'Our brain performance slows down in a state of lower oxygen,' explains Dr Ōkoshi, 'and that can occasionally cause drunk-like symptoms, such as dulling our judgement. When you drink alcohol in such a state, it affects you more, and you feel like you are getting drunk quicker. But this is nothing to do with higher blood alcohol concentration or accelerated absorption of alcohol.

'It might not sound like a big deal if you just get drunk quicker, but for those who have any form of vascular disease, such as heart disease, or diabetes, these conditions can be aggravated. So you need to be very careful.'

The dangers of drinking and dropping off

Dr Ōkoshi actually wore a pulse oximeter on a flight from Tokyo to Bangkok in order to record the changes in levels of oxygen saturated concentration. It showed that the average oxygen saturated content during the flight was 92.8 per cent, a constant state of low oxygen. But from time to time it dropped below 90 per cent, the threshold for hypoxemia danger levels.

Changes in oxygen saturation during flight

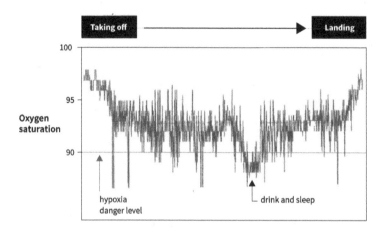

The changes in oxygen saturated concentration levels during a flight between Tokyo and Bangkok. This is data Doctor Ōkoshi himself measured taking a pulse oximeter onboard.

If you study the graph, you will see that the figures plummet in the middle of the flight, spending a while in the hypoxemia danger zone. I asked Dr Ōkoshi what was going on then, and he told me: 'I was asleep, after a few glasses of wine.

'During sleep, even a healthy person can experience shallow breathing, so the oxygen levels get even lower. Meanwhile, alcohol intake blunts the body's reaction to low oxygen. Sleeping after drinking alcohol will augment the low oxygen effects, so it's actually dangerous.'

When I'm on a long-haul flight, I thought the basic idea was to drink alcohol and drop off so my body could have a rest, but far from resting my body, I was putting it in danger!

To make matters worse, in order to get tipsy and fall asleep quickly, I used to drink something with a high ABV content, like a straight whisky or brandy. I feel so stupid now . . . !

Other researchers have investigated blood oxygen concentration levels before and after alcohol intake at a low altitude (171m above sea level) and a high location (3000m). It was confirmed in both places that oxygen concentration levels drop after the ingestion of alcohol. In other words, drinking alcohol contributes to the body's reduced oxygen levels.[26]

Cabin humidity is 20 per cent – super dry!

Dr Ōkoshi warns that it's not only the low oxygen levels that are dangerous.

'On top of that,' he continues, 'you need to keep an eye on dehydration due to the dryness in the cabin. Alcohol has a diuretic effect, which aggravates dehydration and can lead to health problems, such as the so-called economy-class syndrome (thrombosis).

'The inside of an aircraft is extremely dry. Within half an hour of take-off, the humidity percentage drops into the 30s, and then almost down to 20 per cent. Those figures are less than half of acceptable humidity, which is usually something between 40 and 70 per cent. If you're in that dryness, and you're drinking alcohol, which has a diuretic effect, your blood is going to run out of its water supply. The blood thickens, and increases the risk of blood clots. Even if you aren't drinking, you are already more susceptible to blood clots because you are stuck in the same position for a long time during the flight.

'This is why mid-air drinking can trigger economy-class syndrome. To avoid it, the best thing you can do is avoid alcohol. That applies in particular to people with vascular diseases, such as heart disease, or lifestyle illnesses. Also any women taking pills that carry a blood clot warning should be extra careful.'

---

26 Roeggla, G. et.al. 'Effect of Alcohol on Acute Ventilatory Adaptation to Mild Hypoxia at Moderate Altitude' in *Annals of Internal Medicine* 1995; 122: 925–927.

To be sure, the airplane cabin can be extraordinarily dry. My skin and eyes get dried out. If you're in such a situation, a drinker is going to feel thirsty, and immediately think that beer will be the answer, but alcohol is only going to make it worse. It certainly won't help you rehydrate.

Even the airline websites say this. Look closely enough and you'll find them warning that 'alcohol has a diuretic effect, so more urine will be discharged, reducing the water content of the blood and increasing the risk of blood clots'.

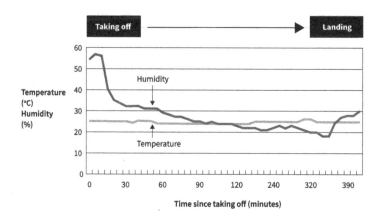

Changes in humidity and temperature in the cabin during flight

Changes in humidity and temperature in the cabin during a flight between Tokyo and Bangkok. The temperature is maintained at about 24 degrees centigrade using air conditioning. Meanwhile, the humidity drops to 30 per cent level half an hour after taking off, then two hours after that it becomes roughly 20 per cent due to the low humidity of air taken in from outside.

How much can we drink?

But, drinkers being drinkers, even with this information, they are liable to want a drink anyway. So if we are stuck on a flight, how much can we drink?

'I would rather you avoid alcohol altogether,' says Dr Ōkoshi, 'but if you really must drink, drink less. This is only a guideline, but it might be wise to stop at about half the usual amount. Also, drinks with a high ABV, such as whisky and brandy, will affect you more if you drink them straight or on the rocks, so mix them with water. What you really need to watch out for is carbonated drinks, such as beer and sparkling wine. It's best to avoid them, because the air expands inside the stomach and intestines during the flight, and will make you feel gassy.'

I asked if it was okay to have some drinks before the flight instead of on it, and I got a telling-off from Dr Ōkoshi.

'It's out of the question,' he said, 'to get drunk in one environment, and then throw yourself into another one where the air pressure and humidity will change.'

Yes, I suppose that the effects would be the same. Silly question.

Drink 100ml of water per hour

Are there any other points we should note, apart from suppressing alcohol intake? Dr Ōkoshi recommends frequent hydration.

'Taking in water is very important,' he says. 'Including the water content of any food you might eat, try to ingest about 100ml of water per hour. It varies from person to person, but 2ml of water per kilo of body weight is an appropriate amount. So if you are 50kg, you should take about 100ml. If you are 100kg, I recommend you take 200ml, so twice as much. Before you get thirsty, drink water frequently.'

He also has some advice against blood clots.

'Do light exercises, such as bending and stretching your legs on a long flight.' For women, it can be effective to wear compressing stockings. Also, if you have a leg in a plaster cast, you could talk to your doctor beforehand about getting some anti-coagulants prescribed.

'I know I've put the frighteners on you, but there is nothing to fear,' he says. 'The most important thing to be aware of is that you are in a different environment from being on the ground. And bearing that in mind, it doesn't take as much alcohol as usual to get you plastered. From a doctor's point of view, I would advise you to start drinking after you get off the plane!'

Drinking used to be one of the things I would look forward to on a long flight, and airline companies used to make serving alcohol a major part of their in-flight activities. But since around the year 2000, there have been increasingly frequent news stories about economy-class syndrome, and airline attitudes to booze have changed. They now offer warnings on their websites about avoiding alcohol intake.

There are many people who travel abroad for long holidays. If you drink so much on the way there that you make yourself ill, you could ruin an otherwise enjoyable trip. Also, if something should happen to the plane, you will compromise your ability to take appropriate action if you are completely blasted. To avoid ruining an expensive trip, try to keep from drinking too much on a plane.

Not just 'Economy class'!?

Economy-class syndrome was originally described as if it only happened to passengers in the cheap seats on an airplane, but it can happen to people in different classes or in different vehicles. Therefore, the Japan Society of Aerospace and Environmental Medicine has suggested 'air travel thrombosis', the term used in Western countries, as being more appropriate.

Why Do We Repeat Ourselves?
Why Do We Repeat Ourselves?
Why . . . ?

Expert Adviser: Ryūsuke Kakigi
National Institute for Physiological Sciences,
National Institutes of Natural Science

Drunken behaviours can be comical and bizarre. When we get drunk, we find ourselves repeating the same thing over and over again, or insisting on a long walk home rather than taking the train. There is a correlation between the brain and alcohol that leads to such unique actions. I asked Ryūsuke Kakigi of National Institute for Physiological Sciences, National Institutes of Natural Science, who is studying the relationship between the human body and the brain, to explain.

'The brain has a blood brain barrier,' he said, 'which blocks harmful substances from the brain. It will only allow fat-soluble materials through, along with items with a molecular weight under 500 Da. Alcohol, which meets both requirements, can make it easily pass the barrier and temporarily paralyse certain brain functions, which can bring out all sorts of behaviours.' [27]

---

27 The molecular weight of ethanol, categorised as primary alcohol, is 46.07.

'There are three areas most affected,' continues Professor Kakigi. 'The frontal lobe, the cerebellum and the hippocampus. The frontal lobe manages thoughts and reasoning, the cerebellum controls motor function, and the hippocampus stores memory. Bizarre behaviours unique to drunks, which are beyond the imagination of sober people, are caused by malfunctions in these areas.'

To be frank, a paralysed frontal lobe makes you bolder

'The frontal lobe is the brain's guardian of reason – it maintains our rational behaviour. But once we consume alcohol, the frontal lobe is gradually released from guard duty, and as a result, this control function eases off. You know how people get intoxicated, and then start making derogatory remarks, revealing secrets and boasting? In the early stages, there are theories that suggest this is caused by a stimulant action of brain hormones, such as dopamine and adrenalin. But if they start to say something they would never have dared to utter before, it's a typical indicator that the frontal lobe has been compromised.'

Effects vary from person to person, but talking in a loud voice, making lewd comments, insisting on a long walk home . . . all these are caused by a compromised frontal lobe. The more you drink, the more the frontal lobe loses its hold on your behaviour. Sudden, intense, hectoring conversations are also part of it. The frontal lobe is released by alcohol, and that makes people chattier.

But badmouthing and boasting are still only mild symptoms. The drunker you get, the worse your behaviour can become. And that's where the cerebellum gets involved.

The cerebellum controls your balance and fine motor skills, as well as the way you process sensory information.

'When the function of the cerebellum is impeded by alcohol,' says Professor Kakigi, 'we can't maintain the smoothness or accuracy of our motor skills. So people stagger, slur and become unable to perform fine motor skills using their fingertips, such as operating smartphones. This is the "drunk" state we all recognise.'

Show me the way to go home – long-term memory still allows for navigation

Many drinkers experience memory loss. You panic the morning after, wondering if you paid the tab at the second bar. You call a friend who tells you that you were still making sense, and that you did get the bill, but you can't remember any of it. The secret to this phenomenon lies in the hippocampus.

'The hippocampus has two roles,' explains Professor Kakigi. 'One is holding short-term memory, and the other is converting it to long-term memory. Short-term memory is very limited – it's like data you put into your computer without saving it. When a drunk repeats the same story or can't remember if they have paid, it's because they've lost the short-term memory data that tells them they've already done something.'

This is why drunk people repeat the same thing over and over again. But even if you can't remember the conversation you just had, how can you somehow always find the way home, as if you have a satnav built in?

Professor Kakigi says it's down to the long-term memory.

'Long-term memory,' he says, 'also called autobiographical memory or episodic memory, is what stays in your brain for a long time. The journey home can get fixed in your long-term memory by constant repetition, because you take the same route every day. That's why you can somehow find your way home, even if you can't remember getting there.'

Incidents away from home, such as not being able to find the hotel when you are drunk at a holiday resort or on a business trip, are caused by the fact that the journey has yet to be fixed in your long-term memory.

Unravelling the relationship between alcohol and your brain helps explain all sorts of bizarre drunken behaviour. However, it's only the person in question who can laugh it off. The people who have to put up with a drunk's behaviour often don't find it quite so amusing.

If this is sounding familiar to you, then maybe you should be reconsidering your relationship with booze.

Hurl Power – why do we vomit when we get drunk?

Expert Adviser: Naohiro Furukawa
Faculty of Health Science and Technology,
Kawasaki University of Medical Welfare

One thing every drinker wants to avoid is throwing up.

You enjoy a tasty drink, but vomiting will ruin everything. More than anything else, it doesn't help you feel any better. We have experienced it so many times in the past, and feel it acutely, but it's a sad nature of the habitual drinker that we still, occasionally, drink until we're sick.

Most of us have experienced vomiting, whether you are a drinker or not. But how does vomit actually work. I asked Naohiro Furukawa, an expert of the physiological mechanism of vomiting at the Faculty of Health Science and Technology of the Kawasaki University of Medical Welfare.

'There are several processes that lead to vomit,' says Professor Furukawa. 'First of all, you feel nausea, which is to say, you feel sick. At the same time, there's an autonomic reflex, which is the secretion of a large amount of saliva. There's antiperistalsis, as the small intestine pushes its contents back into the stomach, temporarily storing all the vomit and excreta there. Your breathing stops, and a combination of inspiratory muscle contraction and expiratory muscle contraction leads to a strong abdominal pressure, called retching. At the same time, your body closes the upper oesophageal sphincter (the mouth side of the gullet) and the glottis, and the pylorus (the lower part of the stomach that connects to the duodenum), so that nothing can go back into the intestines. Lastly, the body relaxes the upper oesophageal sphincter, and abdominal pressure releases the vomit and excreta from inside the stomach into the mouth. That is the series of processes that lead to vomiting.'

Vomiting: an essential mechanism to sustain life

'Vomiting is one of the most important physiological mechanisms for sustaining life,' says Professor Furukawa. Certainly, if something is going to kill you if you eat it, being able to throw it up is going to save your life.

However, since we don't have much of a chance to study human vomiting, we have to rely on animal studies, which leaves many unsolved mysteries in terms of human physiology.

According to Professor Furukawa, there are six basic causes for vomit. (1) irritation of the abdominal organs, (2) mediation by blood, (3) stimulation of vestibular sensation, (4) smell, taste or visual input, (5) mental stimulus, and (6) central nervous stimulus. Among these, vomiting caused by alcohol falls under the second category.

Patience is bad for the body! Vomit when you feel like it

'When you drink an excessive amount of alcohol,' says Professor Furukawa, 'the blood concentration of acetaldehyde exceeds the threshold level, and it sends the signal to the place called the chemoreceptor trigger zone in the area postrema of the brain's medulla oblongata. Then, we believe that a signal is sent to the vomiting centre through the solitary nucleus that is involved in oropharynx reflex, taste, and abdominal organ sense. When you drink too much and vomit, it is a signal that "the body is facing an emergency", so just follow your natural physiological reaction and let yourself throw up.'

Some drinkers try to tough it out, trying not to throw up because they don't want to cause a scene (or waste a good drink). But that's bad for the body.

Causes of vomit: the six main factors

1	**abdominal organ irritation** Caused by toxic substance intake, food poisoning, abdominal disease, a blow to the abdomen, radiation exposure to the abdomen, etc.
2	**mediated by blood** Caused by drugs, bacterial toxins, nicotine, gas, alcohol, metabolites, etc.
3	**vestibular sensation stimulation** Caused by travel sickness, Ménière's disease, etc.
4	**smell, taste, visual input** Caused by an irritating smell, bad taste, colours that raise aversion, rotating or shaking videos, etc.
5	**mental input** Caused by suppression of emotions, strong discomfort, fear, stress, trauma, etc.
6	**central nervous stimulation** Caused by brain disease, such as increased intracranial pressure, cerebral haemorrhage, brain tumour, or subarachnoid haemorrhage

Don't stick your fingers down your throat. It's bad for you

Professor Furukawa cautions against trying to help yourself along by sticking your fingers down your throat.

'As I said, vomiting is like an ultimate life support system, and it's taxing for the body. The vomit and excreta include gastric acid and bile that can melt fat and damage the mucus in the alimentary canal. Once you've thrown up, you can get the sensation of something sour stuck in your throat, which usually indicates that the gastric acid has done some damage to your gullet. We believe that the large amount of saliva that gets discharged before vomiting is designed to protect the gullet from gastric acid and bile. However, if you force yourself to throw up before the body is properly ready to, it could cause further damage to the gullet. You should avoid forcing yourself to throw up repeatedly unless you have no other choice but to discharge excess alcohol.'

The complex process of throwing up

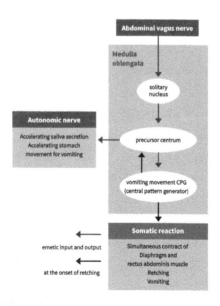

The signal from the vagus nerve in the abdomen is taken to the medulla oblongata, which induces the physical reaction to cause vomit. 'Vomiting movement CPG' is 'a program in the centrum, or neural networks' (Furukawa). (Adapted from Naohiro Furukawa, 'Ōto Yūhatsu no Chūsū Shinkei Kikō: Ōto Undō ni Senkō suru Zenchō Genshō wo Yūhatsu suru Chūsū no Teishō (Central neural mechanism for inducing vomiting)' in *Hikaku Seirise Kagaku*, Volume 16, Issue 3, 1999, 171-179.)

But in that case, what should we do when we feel like throwing up but can't?

'There's some scientific evidence,' says Professor Furukawa, 'that an easy way to induce vomiting if you are feeling nauseous is to hold your breath and sniff something with a strong smell, for example perfume or kimchi. You will be sure to get sick. However, they are not necessarily always around when you need them, so the easiest thing to do would be to drink a few glasses of water to stimulate your stomach to encourage vomiting.'

Avoid vomiting in the bath after drinking

'There is one kind of vomiting that is even more taxing on the body,' says Professor Furukawa, 'and that's throwing up when you are drunk in the bath.

'If you get into a hot bath while heavily drunk, it will increase the blood circulation, which can lead to vomiting. This is just my personal view, but I think it can make you vomit without warning, because the alcohol has paralysed your brain function, dulling the automatic reflexes that would otherwise, say, discharge extra saliva. As a result, such sudden vomiting can cause oesophageal tearing, and in an extreme case, could lead to internal bleeding.'

So, if you are falling-down drunk and think it might be a good idea to sweat it out in a hot bath, that's apparently extremely dangerous. 'Particularly when you are very drunk,' says Professor Furukawa, 'it's wise to wait until the next morning to have a bath.'

Danger sign: nothing but gastric acid

The way to avoid nausea is similar to the way you avoid other ill effects (see page 2). For example, you can eat protein, such as cheese, before you start drinking, in order to delay the stomach's absorption of alcohol.

Should you have nothing in your stomach, and find yourself repeatedly throwing up nothing but gastric acid, then it could be that your body is sending you a danger sign.

'That could mean that you have acute alcohol poisoning,' says Professor Furukawa, 'so I recommend you go straight to A&E.' If your vomiting does not stop, don't try to diagnose yourself.

Nobody wants to end up in the hospital for excessive drinking. Having to seek medical attention should be the last resort. Let's learn how to drink without being bewitched by the magical powers of alcohol.

Exercise for Drunks – can we really 'train' ourselves to drink more?

Expert Adviser: Shinichi Asabe
Jichi Medical University Saitama Medical Center

'We can train ourselves to drink more.'

Many of us have heard this old wives' tale, particularly from older classmates forcing us to go out on the town with them in our college days. I'm living proof of it, since I certainly seemed to be able to hold my booze better, the more I did it. But there are also people who don't seem to be able to train themselves up, and end up endlessly repeating an unpleasant experience.

What determines whether you can drink a lot? I asked Mr Shinichi Asabe from the Jichi Medical University Saitama Medical Center, a liver expert.

It's all in the genes

Your ability to drink a little or a lot is determined by your genetic heritage.

'If drinking makes you feel bad,' says Dr Asabe, 'the culprit is the acetaldehyde generated by the breakdown of alcohol. The acetaldehyde is broken down in turn by aldehyde dehydrogenase, but the efficiency of that activity is genetically determined. If you have two "heavyweight" genes, you can drink a lot because you break down the acetaldehyde quickly. If you have two "lightweight" genes, you're the kind of person who can't drink a lot, because the acetaldehyde builds up too quickly.' (See page 76)

So your ability to put it away or get swiftly tipsy is determined in the womb. If you have heavyweight parents, you can drink like a fish, while if your parents couldn't handle alcohol, you probably can't, either.

'Race is also a factor in your ability to hold your drink,' continues Dr Asabe. 'Nearly 100 per cent of Caucasians and black people have the gene combination that makes them heavyweight drinkers. But among the Mongoloid races (including the Japanese and Chinese), about 50 per cent are heavyweights, 10 per cent are lightweights, and the rest have the ability to learn how to drink more.

'Interestingly, that last 40 per cent who have both heavy and lightweight genes start off extremely lightweight, but are able to handle alcohol more by becoming accustomed to it. The more chances they have to drink alcohol, the more heavyweight they become.'

Dr Asabe says that quite a few people think that they cannot drink, even though they have heavyweight genes. An easy way to learn your own alcohol tolerance is to try the patch test mentioned on page 81 of this book.

Training the enzyme that metabolises drugs

'Your acetaldehyde dehydrogenase can be enhanced by repeatedly metabolising alcohol,' says Dr Asabe. 'The process also enhances an enzyme called cytochrome P450 (CYP3A4), which is involved in the process of metabolising alcohol.' [28]

---

28 There are many varieties of cytochromes, but those involved in metabolising alcohol are thought to be CYP2E1 and CYP3A4.

Most of the CYP3A4 in the body is found in the liver, where it helps break down chemicals. When the body is spurred to produce more of it, people feel less sick, and their faces flush less when they increase their alcohol intake. Sadly, it's impossible to test for a statistical ranking of your CYP3A4 levels, but if you feel like you can tolerate a higher level of alcohol than you used to, CYP3A4 probably has something to do with it.

However, if you don't drink for a while, the activity of both enzymes will slow again, and even a small amount of alcohol will make you drunk. Dr Asabe himself is one of those people who is not a heavyweight, but had heavyweight potential. He experimented on himself, staying away from alcohol for a whole month in order to allow his acetaldehyde dehydrogenase and CYP3A4 levels to drop down from a relatively high level of activity. After a dry month, he found that he very easily got drunk.

'Acetaldehyde dehydrogenase activity varies from person to person,' adds Dr Asabe, 'so you shouldn't force yourself to "train". The kind of person who gets addicted to alcohol isn't one of the heavyweights, but one of that 40 per cent group that only has heavyweight potential.' If you drink habitually, you may start to think that you are a heavyweight, but instead you just increase the amount gradually until, in a worst-case scenario, you have become dependent on alcohol. Once you get to that stage, being a heavyweight is the least of your problems – you need expert help.

Even if you do train yourself to hold more drink, that will be no use to you if it makes you ill. Do not force yourself. See how you are feeling on the day, and never drink so much that you will get a hangover. This is the secret of enjoying a long and moderate drinking life.

If you train your CYP3A4, medicine can become less effective!

CYP3A4 determines your alcohol tolerance, but you should be aware that there is a cost to enhancing its activity.

When CYP3A4's activity increases, it also increases the speed with which any active ingredients might be metabolised, not merely alcohol. As a result, you might not get the expected effects from certain chemicals, including drugs used to combat hypertension (adalert), benzodiazepine sleeping pills (e.g. halcion), anti-coagulants like warfarin, and cholesterol-lowering drugs like statins.

If you routinely take these drugs, you need to take extra care.

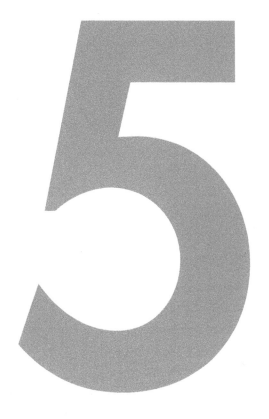

The Science Part – recent research into alcohol and illness

Bum Deal – how drinking raises the risk of colorectal cancer

Expert Adviser: Tetsuya Mizoue
Center for Clinical Sciences,
National Center for Global Health and Medicine

All drinkers are sure to worry about cancer. After all, cancers are the largest cause of death among many populations, the Japanese included. The probability of getting cancer at some point in one's life is as high as 63 per cent for men and 47 per cent for women. And as you may know already, one of the major factors that increases the risk of cancer is drinking.

It's particularly well-known that drinking increases the risk of getting laryngeal or oesophageal cancer. An acquaintance of mine with a penchant for whisky on the rocks probably has that to blame for his oesophageal cancer.

Colorectal cancer hits people in their prime

Of all cancers, colorectal cancer has to be the one that worries middle-aged businesspeople most. According to data published by National Cancer Center Japan in August 2016, the disease rate by locus shows that colorectal cancer is the biggest cause of death in Japanese women, and the third biggest cause for Japanese men. The onset rate goes up when people reach their fifties, so yes, it affects those in the prime of life.

And since fifty is looming for me, I can't let this one pass. Come to think of it, I find myself hearing more and more stories from my fellow drinkers that their latest health screening found polyps in their colon, and they've had early-stage colorectal cancer removed. And there are quite a few stories of celebrities dying from colorectal cancer.

I used to think that colorectal cancer was caused by a diet heavy in meat and fat. There was a widely circulated media story in 2015, stating that red meat and processed meat both increase the risk of colorectal cancer. But it turns out those were not the only probable causes.

I'd also heard that drinking is a major influence on colorectal cancer, but is that true? And if it is, why does drinking make it worse? I put these questions to Tetsuya Mizoue from the Center for Clinical Sciences, National Center for Global Health and Medicine.

Colorectal cancer has claimed 50,000 lives in Japan!

'We used to think of colorectal cancer as a Western problem,' says Dr Mizoue, 'but it is becoming a major problem in Japan. The number of fatalities from colorectal cancer in Japan has now reached about 50,000.'

Is this because of our adoption of a Western-style diet?

'As you suggest, the change to our lifestyle has a lot to do with it. The Western diet, which is to say, food that includes a lot of meat and fat, has an adverse impact on Japanese people with their long intestines. As you know, the risks of red meat and processed meats have been flagged up and widely discussed. But they are not the only factors that increase the risk of this cancer. It's not as widely known, but drinking is also a major factor in increasing the risk of the disease.'

Drinking is certain to raise the risk

The National Cancer Center Japan has evaluated the causal relationship between cancer and the lifestyle of Japanese people. Based on the latest research both from Japan and overseas, it publishes an overall risk evaluation and individual locus cancer report on its website: a list of cancer risks and protective factors. According to this evaluation, the only *certain* factor that contributes to colorectal cancer is drinking. The next factor in line is obesity, but that is only *almost* certain. So how much does alcohol contribute to the risk of colorectal cancer?

Dr Mizoue's research group analysed the data from 200,000 people in five cohort studies, evaluating the relationship between Japanese drinking habits and the risk of colorectal cancer. The results were published in a specialist journal in 2008. It concluded that: 'excessive drinking among both men and women increases the overall risk of colorectal cancer, colon cancer and rectal cancer. It is particularly notable for men.'

The bowel covers a large area – the rectum is the bit near the anus, and then the colon extends upward from the curved area above the rectum (the sigmoid colon). The increased risk of cancer applies to both areas.

Looking at Dr Mizoue's analysis men who drink 23–45.9g, 46–68.9g, 69–91.9g and over 92g of pure alcohol a day have, respectively, 1.4 times, 2.0 times, 2.2 times and 3.0 times the risk when compared to a non-drinking group. There is a demonstrable risk, running in proportion to the amount of alcohol someone drinks. The cases among women are not as notable, but those who drank more than 23g of pure alcohol per day had 1.6 times the risk of those who did not drink at all.

To be honest, I had not expected the effect of drinking to be so obvious. This is a shocking revelation for drinkers who worry about colorectal cancer. And 23g of alcohol is the equivalent of a single cup of saké – that's not much for a daily tippler.

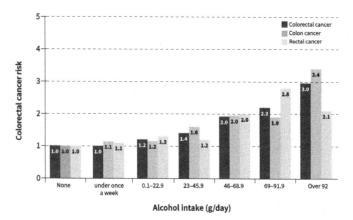

Correlation between alcohol intake and colorectal cancer (men)

The risk of colorectal cancer increases along with alcohol intake (relative risk when the risk of the group with non-drinkers as set as one). This suggests when alcohol intake is increased by 15g, the risk of colorectal cancer increases by 10 per cent. (Tetsuya Mizoue, Manami Inoue, Kenji Wakai, et al., 'Alcohol Drinking and Colorectal Cancer in Japanese: A Pooled Analysis of Results from Five Cohort Studies' in *American Journal of Epidemiology*, Volume 167, Issue 12, 15 June 2008, 1397-1406.)

Why does drinking cause colorectal cancer?

Dr Mizoue has also analysed the correlation between alcohol intake and colorectal cancer in two other groups – Japanese people and Westerners. According to that data, when Westerners increase their alcohol intake, there is a gentle rise in risk, but when Japanese people do the same thing, the risk jumps up sharply for them. Is this because Japanese people have a lower tolerance for alcohol?

'As a race, the Japanese people have a lower alcohol tolerance,' admits Dr Mizoue. 'For Westerners, with a high alcohol tolerance, the risk of colorectal cancer doesn't increase until they start drinking more than two cups of saké a day, whereas by that point, the Japanese are already at between 1.4 and 1.8 the level of risk.'

So we need to accept that there is a specific racial difference. Bad news for the Japanese.

But what is the mechanism that leads to colorectal cancer?

'We don't know for sure, yet, what actually makes it happen,' says Dr Mizoue, 'but the most likely cause is the toxicity of acetaldehyde. Tests have found that acetaldehyde, produced during the metabolising of alcohol, is a carcinogen. If you routinely drink a large amount of alcohol, or if you are one of those people who get red-faced, then you are prolonging your exposure to acetaldehyde, and that could put you at a higher risk.

'However, there's been recent research that looks into the relationship between gene types and colorectal cancer, and it didn't necessarily show up any clear connections. So the current medical opinion is that your genetic heritage doesn't have much to do with colorectal cancer. It's more about the way that acetaldehyde generated by alcohol processing prevents the body from absorbing and using folic acid.'

The bowel is divided into the 'rectum' and 'colon'

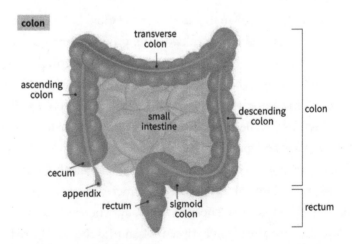

'Rectal cancer' in the rectum near the anus and 'sigmoid colon cancer' in the sigmoid colon located just above the rectum account for 70 per cent of all colorectal cancers.

**Japanese drinkers have a higher risk of colorectal cancer
than their Western counterparts**

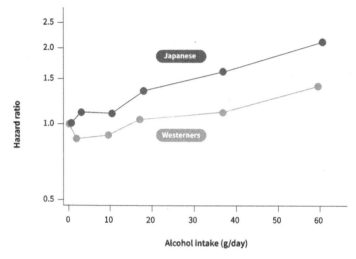

Comparison of correlation between alcohol intake and the risk of colorectal cancer
for Japanese and Westerners (Tetsuya Mizoue, Manami Inoue, Kenji Wakai, et al.,
'Alcohol Drinking and Colorectal Cancer in Japanese: A Pooled Analysis of Results
from Five Cohort Studies' in *American Journal of Epidemiology*, Volume 167, Issue
12, 15 June 2008, 1397-1406.)

Actively take in folic acid

'Folic acid is a type of B-vitamin,' explains Dr Mizoue, 'and as the
name suggests, you can find it in leafy vegetables. It's an important
nutrient in the process of cell synthesis and cell repair, and it's
essential for the synthesis of DNA with genetic information in cells.
But as I said, acetaldehyde prevents the intestines from absorbing
folic acid. That is believed to prevent the body from synthesising
and repairing cells, which can lead to damaged genes – an early
stage of colorectal cancer.'

So although the precise mechanism isn't clear, it seems that folic
acid may have something to do with cancer prevention. I felt that
this was offering me a small amount of hope. Does this mean that

if I routinely take folic acid supplements, I can prevent colorectal cancer even if I keep on drinking?

'Unfortunately, we can't say for sure,' replies Dr Mizoue. 'It might be that consuming a large amount of folic acid would reduce the risk of colorectal cancer, but the factors that cause colorectal cancer are very complex. It's not like lung cancer, for which smoking is a clear cause. Having said that, there's no harm in actively consuming folic acid to make up the deficit. You can find it in green vegetables like broccoli, spinach and Japanese mustard spinach, as well as in citrus fruits. I recommend taking folic acid in the form of fresh food, not as a supplement.'

It is better to avoid excessive drinking

For Dr Mizoue, the critical factor is the amount that we drink.

'As you could see from the graphs,' he says, 'the risk of colorectal cancer rises with alcohol intake. So, first of all, you shouldn't go over 23 to 24.9g a day of pure alcohol – that's one or two cups of saké, or a 500ml bottle of beer. That's your baseline.'

And we are back again to our old friend, the moderate amount.

Dr Mizoue adds that dietary fibre is also a key.

'I recommend that you actively consume grain-based dietary fibre. In the past, we used to think that vegetable fibre, such as burdock root, was good, but recent research has suggested that the fibre contained in grains, such as rice and wheat, is more effective. It's good to mix plain white rice with other grains. And you should consume food that is calcium-rich, such as milk.'

I'm sure that many of you are already having brown rice and barley as part of an everyday diet. It's great that everyday ingredients, rather than something odd and special, are effective in this case.

Dr Mizoue also warns that obesity increases the risk of colorectal cancer.

'Make sure your BMI doesn't go over 25,' he says. 'For that reason, you should get into the habit of 150 minutes a week of exercise.'

Obesity is the cause of a number of conditions, not merely cancer. If you are diagnosed as overweight, you need to take care. The 150 minutes a week that Dr Mizoue recommends amounts to just over 20 minutes a day. You can achieve that without too much effort with just a little bit of application, such as getting off a stop early and walking the rest of the way home, or consciously taking the stairs instead of using the elevator.

There are more cases of colorectal cancer today than there were in the past. It's no wonder that so many people worry about it, but Dr Mizoue points out: 'If you catch it in an early enough stage, you have a high chance of recovering from it. So early diagnosis is the key. Once you hit your forties, get a colorectal cancer check once a year.'

Don't worry too much, but do get regular check-ups and watch your daily diet. Then you can enjoy drinking for many years to come.

St Pancreas – pancreatitis might mean you have to stop drinking altogether

Expert Adviser: Kyōko Shimizu
Department of Internal Medicine and Gastroenterology,
Tokyo Women's Medical University

Drinkers seem to be most preoccupied with their liver – that hard-working organ that breaks down alcohol. So they are always checking their medical results for liver function scores, such as gamma-GTP and ALT. They have 'liver holidays' because they care about their livers, and they think that everything will be fine, as long as they look after their livers. But . . . in fact, there is another organ that they should take care with, perhaps even more than their liver, and that's the pancreas. It's often known as a 'silent organ' (as is the liver), and plays an important role in digestion.

To find out just how important, I asked Kyōko Shimizu from the Department of Internal Medicine and Gastroenterology, Tokyo Women's Medical University, about the relationship between alcohol and the pancreas.

The pancreas is an important organ with an influence on obesity and diabetes

'There are two main functions for the pancreas,' she says. 'One is exocrine function, to secrete enzymes that digest protein, fats and carbohydrates. The other is the endocrine function, to release hormones, such as insulin and glucagon, which control blood sugar levels.'

The low-carb diet has been popular recently, and many of you might have heard its key word: insulin. Insulin is also the stuff that people with type-2 diabetes have to inject, as their body does not produce enough of it to control their blood sugar levels.

Compared to other organs, the pancreas might be less familiar, but for us drinkers, it plays an important role in the digestive system, alongside more familiar organs, such as the liver, the stomach and the intestines.

Even after acute symptoms subside, is it not completely cured?

When it comes to alcohol and the pancreas, the drinkers' deepest concern is pancreatitis. Over the last few years, it's been news that several well-known Japanese comedians developed the disease. All of them were men in their late thirties or forties.

'Pancreatitis is literally an inflamed pancreas,' explains Dr Shimizu. 'Acute pancreatitis comes with subjective symptoms, such as severe pain in the upper abdomen or the back, and nausea.

'There's acute pancreatitis and chronic pancreatitis, but even if you develop acute pancreatitis and the symptoms subside, it does not mean that you are completely cured. Most of those who develop alcoholic pancreatitis already have chronic pancreatitis due to routine drinking over a long period of time, and when daily alcoholic intake increases for a while during, for example, the party season, alcohol can trigger an "acute" episode. In other words, when the symptoms appear, it is often the case that the pancreas already has been chronically inflamed.'

Even in an acute case, a serious case of pancreatitis can lead to multiple organ failure. Why do such symptoms occur?

Main cases for chronic pancreatitis

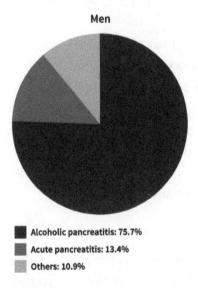

Men

■ Alcoholic pancreatitis: 75.7%
■ Acute pancreatitis: 13.4%
□ Others: 10.9%

Of all the causes of pancreatitis, alcoholic pancreatitis accounts for 75.7 per cent in men. (Ministry of Health, Labour and Welfare, Research Group for Intractable Diseases and Refractory Pancreatic Diseases, Nationwide Survey on Chronic Pancreatitis, 2002.)

'Firstly,' says Dr Shimizu, 'the main symptom of pancreatitis is the abnormal secretion of pancreatic fluid, including the digestive enzyme trypsin, which breaks down proteins. In a normal state, trypsin would reach the duodenum in an inactive state, and only become active when it mixes with enterokinase, an enzyme secreted from the small intestine, to digest food. However, various factors, including alcohol, make trypsin active in the pancreas causing it to start "digesting" the organ itself. That is what pancreatitis is. In a severe case of acute pancreatitis, a wide area of the pancreas undergoes necrosis, releasing a large amount of active substance to the whole body, which can lead to multiple organ failure, then, unfortunately, to death. Continuous inflammation of the pancreas is chronic pancreatitis, which destroys normal tissues over many years. Because they undergo fibrosis (shrinkage), this can cause digestion and absorption abnormalities. Also, lowering the body's endocrine function will increase the risk of diabetes.'

The risk of pancreatitis increases with the accumulation of ethanol!

According to the reports from the Research Group for Intractable Diseases and Refractory Pancreatic Diseases, sponsored by the Japanese Ministry of Health, Labour and Welfare, the main cause of pancreatitis is alcohol, which accounts for 67.5 per cent of cases in men and women. If we take men as a group in their own right, the rate of cases caused by alcohol goes up to an extremely high 75.7 per cent. Other causes can be gallstones and spontaneous pancreatitis with unknown cause, but they are nothing compared to alcohol. The common thing about the comedians I referred to earlier, who all developed pancreatitis, is that all of them were known to like a drink or two. Considering such facts, it is clear that the drinkers who cannot do without alcohol are liable to be in an inseparable relationship with pancreatitis.

'It's not about what you drink,' says Dr Shimizu. 'It doesn't matter if it's a spirit or a brew. What's important is the accumulation of ethanol over time. If you spend a decade drinking the equivalent of 80g a day, the risk increases.' That's two litres of beer or four cups of saké, not a huge amount for a heavy drinker; for women, the same kind of risk arises with about 60 per cent as much.

'We believe that this is the reason that so many people develop pancreatitis in their thirties and forties,' says Dr Shimizu. 'Also, recently there has been more of a focus on the genes related to the development of pancreatitis. It is believed that mutated genes could increase the risk, and that some people end up physically prone to develop the disease, regardless of alcohol intake.'

It's difficult to repair damage to the pancreas

The key is, as ever, to review your lifestyle and the amount of alcohol you drink.

'Basically, try not to drink a huge amount of alcohol,' she says. 'Keep to a moderate amount of 20g daily in pure alcohol conversion. Smoking is also a factor in pancreatitis and pancreatic cancer, so if you are smoker, I advise you to stop. The next thing is to keep a regular lifestyle and try to release stress. And in order to reduce the burden on pancreatic function, it is important to take moderate exercise and avoid becoming obese. For diet, I recommend avoiding highly fatty foods that place a burden on the pancreas, and actively try to enjoy a traditional Japanese diet, like simmered dishes and grilled fish.'

Mortality factors for patients with chronic pancreatitis

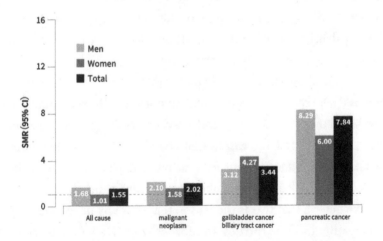

Standardised mortality ratios for each mortality factor of pancreatitis patients during the follow-up was calculated based on the nationwide vital statistics of 1998. For both men and women, death caused by pancreatic cancer is higher than for the general public (Ministry of Health, Labour and Welfare, the Research Group for Intractable Diseases and Refractory Pancreatic Diseases, Nationwide Survey on Chronic Pancreatitis, 2002).

Such advice might be easy to consider for the general public, but for the hard-core drinker, the words 'moderate amount' tend to become a distant memory as soon as they are out on the town. However, we shouldn't take pancreatic damage lightly.

'Once you develop pancreatitis,' explains Dr Shimizu, 'it is really rather difficult to restore it to its original state. Advanced pancreatitis increases the risk of pancreatic cancer, which is difficult to spot, and hard for current medicine to cure.'

Hardly any symptoms until it's too late

Why is it difficult to prevent and find pancreatic disease, even with modern medicine?

'Because the pancreas is located behind the stomach,' she says. 'People think that if they experience pain, it must be coming from the stomach, which can lead to pancreatic diseases being slow to diagnose. Unlike the stomach or colon, it's not possible to see it directly with an endoscopy. For something like your lungs, we can't see them directly, but we have other devices, like a helical CT, that can investigate any problems. But the best we can do with the pancreas is to evaluate the amylase levels in a blood test. Even with an abdominal ultrasound, the pancreas is in a hard-to-see place, so if we suspect a pancreatic disease, we have to carry out a more detailed test like a contrast-enhanced CT or an MRI. As the pancreas is what we call a "silent organ", you rarely experience any subjective symptoms until the disease is quite advanced, so it is easy not to notice it.'

And once you have developed pancreatitis, it's too late to just swear you'll drink moderately from now on.

'Speaking as an expert,' says Dr Shimizu, 'I wouldn't have any choice but to advise you to stop drinking for the rest of your life.'

Abstinence might sound like the worst possible sentence for a drinker, but thereafter you would be living under the threat of pancreatitis turning into full-blown pancreatic cancer. In fact, looking at the standardised mortality ratio, which is the mortality rate compared to the general public, the number for those who go on to die from pancreatic cancer after developing pancreatitis is a ratio of 7.84, the highest of all.

With an organ like the pancreas, which, unlike the liver, does not have a restorative function, we are obliged to use what we already have, carefully. It's very difficult for drinkers to control the urge to drink, but compared to a life without any alcohol at all, which would you prefer?

If you wish to live with alcohol, in small amounts for a long time, then don't forget to take care of your pancreas.

Like It or Lump It – breast cancer and alcohol

Expert Adviser: Seigo Nakamura
Breast Surgical Oncology,
Showa University School of Medicine

In 2015, the celebrity Akira Hokuto announced that she had been diagnosed with breast cancer, which raised the awareness of the disease more than ever. Following her announcement, more Japanese women tried to get breast cancer screening, and for a while, it was difficult to make an appointment with the Breast Surgical Oncology department.

I do get an annual screening, but at the time, even though my results were negative, I became worried and my husband suggested I should do the screening again.

Disease rate of breast cancer is rocketing

Breast cancer starts in the mammary glands. In 70 to 80 per cent of cases, it is thought that the cancer is stimulated by the female hormone oestrogen . These days, menstruation tends to start earlier and menopause is getting later, so we are exposed to oestrogen longer. With that as a background, the rate of breast cancer is increasing.

In fact, if we compare the data from 1980 and 2003, the disease rate is clearly up, moreover it's particularly notable in people aged forty and up, especially after menopause. According to the data in 2015, the number of Japanese people with breast cancer was 89,000, which more than quadruples the number in the 1980s.

Breast cancer is no longer a rare disease. And the scary thing is that there is a powerful correlation between breast cancer and alcohol intake.

I have talked with my female friends about breast cancer and drinking, but most of them had no idea. Hmm, most of these ladies are drinking alcohol without knowing that there is a risk of the disease.

I asked Seigo Nakamura, chairman of the Japanese Breast Cancer Society and professor at Shōwa University School of Medicine, for his advice.

Drinking increases the risk of developing breast cancer

'Alcohol increases the risk of developing breast cancer,' says Professor Nakamura. 'We have results from several case control studies, which compared those who drink and those who don't, and every single one of them shows that those who drink alcohol are at a higher risk. And the higher the alcohol intake, the higher the disease rate of breast cancer is said to be.'

So there it is – the more you drink, the higher the risk of breast cancer. For ladies who like to drink, that is not 'somebody else's problem'.

Evidence gathered by the World Cancer Research Fund (WCRF) and the American Institute for Cancer Research (AICR) also shows that the risk is judged to be 'probable'. This is the second highest level of the five possible grades: *convincing, probable, limited-suggestive, limited but inconclusive,* and *substantial effect on risk unlikely.* It looks like the effect alcohol has on breast cancer is extraordinary.

'The report published by the WCRF in 2007 also said: "there is strong evidence that alcoholic drinks are the cause of pre- and post-menopausal breast cancer",' adds Professor Nakamura. 'The increase in the risk is 6 to 10 per cent, which is not that high, but there is no doubt that alcohol *does* increase the risk.'

A multi-purpose cohort study of 50,000 women of forty to sixty-nine years of age, carried out by the National Cancer Center Japan over thirteen years, also shows that 'the greater your alcohol intake, the more likely it is you will suffer from breast cancer'. Among the group of people who drink more than a 'moderate' 150g a week in pure alcohol conversion, the risk is 1.75 times greater compared to those who have never drunk.

Why does alcohol increase the risk of breast cancer?

'There are various factors that cause this,' says Professor Nakamura. 'Alcohol is carcinogenic, and so is acetaldehyde, which is what gets generated when the body breaks alcohol down. There's oxidative stress induced by the metabolising of alcohol, and there's an increase in sex hormones. There's a deficiency in folic acid, which is crucial for DNA synthesis and restoration. All those things. But at the moment, we don't really have a clear reason. It's clear from the cohort study data that the risk of breast cancer goes up if you drink more, but at the moment we haven't determined an accurate set of figures.'

So at the moment, there isn't a clear causal relationship, but there is clear evidence that drinking more increases your risk, somehow. So how much should we drink?

'This is only a guide,' says Professor Nakamura, 'but generally, a cup of saké or a 500ml bottle of beer, or two glasses of wine a day, is what we'd call a limited risk. But there is no clear evidence supporting that, either. As I said, the more you drink, the greater the risk, so be careful not to overindulge.'

What about people with strong alcohol tolerance?

'We don't have a clear idea about the mechanism, so I can only speculate. But because acetaldehyde is one of the causes, there is a chance that people who cannot drink, or people who have a lightweight ability to process alcohol, are at a higher risk.'

Yet another reason why we shouldn't force people who cannot drink to have any alcohol.

You also need to watch out for obesity

As a lady who loves booze, this is all sad to hear, but considering the risk of breast cancer, it's better to keep drinking to a modest amount. But of course, when we are talking about the risk, the real question is the size of the risk. How much should we worry about drinking alcohol?

When I asked Professor Nakamura, with tears in my eyes, if it was better for women to refrain from drinking altogether, he said some words that put me at ease.

'It's true that alcohol increases the risk of breast cancer, but you don't need to worry about it too much. As far as factors go that increase the risk of the disease, the most dangerous is currently thought to be obesity, and another is lack of exercise. Both of these present greater dangers than the danger of alcohol. Also, although drinking is a "certain" risk factor in international studies, we don't actually have enough data to confirm whether that is also true in Japan. Having said that, don't let down your guard and drink too much.'

I saw a ray of sunshine in the darkness, but I flinched at the word 'obesity'. For drinkers who like to snack while they're drinking, that can also be a pressing problem.

'Obesity and breast cancer have a close relationship, and that is especially notable after menopause. After menopause, ovarian function declines and oestrogen (female hormone) reduces, so the risk of breast cancer is believed to be reduced. However, if you are obese, that is another matter. The reason is the aromatase enzyme that exists in the adipose tissue of the mammary glands. Aromatase converts androgen, a sort of male hormone produced from cholesterol, into oestrogen, and aromatase is more active in obese people. In other words, the mammary glands end up making more oestrogen, and that is believed to be a major factor in the post-menopause breast cancer rate increase.'

After menopause, fat can be a major source for oestrogen! Looking around, I cannot say most of my guzzler friends are slim by any standard, and quite a few of them are taking medication for gout or diabetes caused by obesity. And if both the WCRF and AICR are grading obesity as a 'convincing' cause of post-menopause cancer . . . Oh, I should lose some weight . . .

What is the correlation between soy or dairy products and breast cancer?

'One of the reasons for the increased rate of breast cancer,' says Professor Nakamura, 'is that the Japanese have adopted a Westernised diet.' Looking at the Food Balance Sheet published by the Japanese Ministry of Agriculture, Forestry and Fisheries, calories from rice dropped below a quarter of daily food intake in 2003, while calories from animal products, oil and fat quadrupled. The overall calorie intake per day is 300 kilocalories more than it was for the Japanese in 1960. And all the good snacks that come with alcoholic drinks are greasy, high-calorie stuff. We need to keep an eye not only on what we drink, but what we eat alongside it.

Talking about snacks, there is a rumour that the isoflavone contained in soybeans can reduce the recurrence of breast cancer.

Other rumours suggest that dairy products, including cheese, can make you more susceptible to breast cancer. Are they true?

'There are reports that soybeans have a preventative effect,' says Professor Nakamura, 'so eating them will do you no harm. But you shouldn't expect that ingesting a large quantity of soy will somehow reduce your risk. Some people take isoflavone supplements because they think it can reduce the risk of breast cancer, but speaking as a doctor, I wouldn't recommend it. There are arguments both for and against the risk factors of dairy products, but we simply don't have enough evidence either way.'

So, it seems that I should drop the idea of eating something to ward off breast cancer.

Exercise reduces the risk of breast cancer

What Professor Nakamura can recommend, however, is exercise.

'Exercise might reduce your body weight, but it can also reduce the risk of breast cancer,' he says. It doesn't matter if you are pre- or post-menopausal, exercise helps maintain a healthy body weight and prevents obesity. That, in turn, can hold off lifestyle diseases, so if anything, I am coming away from our talk with a resolution to keep fitter.

There's no point in fretting too much about your alcohol intake, but there is no denying that it increases your risk. The keys to reducing that risk are preventing obesity and exercising. Reducing your alcohol intake will help, here, as will not eating too much and looking after your body. To beat breast cancer and maintain health, why don't you start today?

Hairs on Your Chest – does too much drinking reduce male hormones!?

Expert Adviser: Shigeo Horie
Juntendō University Graduate School of Medicine

Just as ladies fret about female hormones, men get a light in their eyes when they hear that something 'helps male hormones'. Sometimes I think . . . no, I pretty much know for sure that men are more sensitive about the word 'hormones' than women are. They think that hormones maketh the man – I suppose they want to boast about their manliness, no matter how old they are. How adorable – any old geezer can be cute in the right light.

What is the relationship between alcohol and male hormones?

Well, let's start with the first male hormone that springs to mind: testosterone. But it's something of a misnomer to call it 'male' at all, because women have testosterone as well. As the name implies, for men, 95 per cent of it is made in the testicles while 5 per cent is made in the adrenal glands. Women get their testosterone from their adrenal glands, too, although some it is manufactured in their fat cells and ovaries.

Testosterone contributes to the development of muscles and bones, and reaches peak secretion at about age twenty, before gradually declining thereafter. Reduction of testosterone is linked to erectile dysfunction and a declining sex drive, but there is more to it than that. Testosterone is often discussed as a hormone connected to 'social performance', as it is vital to both men and women in their attractiveness and societal acceptance.

In fact, when doctors are investigating a potential diagnosis of depression, they may check testosterone levels. Low readings there might suggest a form of depression caused by late-onset hypogonadism, or LOH-syndrome, also known as the male menopause.

Testosterone is a hormone essential to the living of an energetic life, for both men and women. But there are stories circulating on the internet that drinking alcohol can reduce your testosterone levels, which is sure to get the drinkers worried. What is the truth? I put the question to Shigeo Horie, a professor at the Juntendō University Graduate School of Medicine and chairman of the Japanese Society of Men's Health.

No need to worry if you are drinking a normal level

'Basically,' he says, 'there is no direct link between a normal level of drinking and a decline in testosterone levels. In fact, moderate drinking has the effect of actually raising the testosterone level, in both men and women. If you habitually drink a larger amount, then there will be an effect, but you needn't worry as long as you are drinking a reasonable amount. If you exercise before you drink, your testosterone levels will also go up, whether you drink a lot or not.'

Ooh! What wonderful words to hear! Men all over can drink away!

'But,' he adds, uh-oh, 'there is a risk if you drink a lot of beer. It won't affect you if you are someone who just has beer as an aperitif for other drinks, but if you drink beer from start to finish you need to watch out. That's because hops, one of the ingredients in beer, contains a substance called naringenin which acts like a female hormone that can prevent the secretion of testosterone.'

How much beer will do that to you?

'If you drink more than three 500ml cans a night,' says Professor Horie, 'then it might affect you. But if you're worried about it, drink something else. Wine, saké or *shōchū* don't have the same properties.'

Avoid chronic over-drinking

It's a relief to hear that drinking a normal amount will not affect testosterone, but drinking excessively is another matter.

'If you drink excessively,' cautions Professor Horie, 'then any alcohol, not just beer, might reduce your testosterone. Over an extended period of time, the ethanol in alcoholic drinks can damage the cells in the spermary that produce testosterone. Excessive drinking can adversely affect the production of the hormone. Metabolising ethanol reduces your stocks of nicotinamide adenine dinucleotide (NAD), which is the vitamin essential for maintaining the energy balance of the cells in the liver and the spermary. This could be one of the reasons why excessive alcohol can damage the liver.'

Bit of a digression, but Professor Horie says that sperm can be affected by excessive drinking, too. According to him, 'too much alcohol can get the sperm drunk'. And that can affect the foetus, too.

Obesity is a greater danger than alcohol

Professor Horie says that weight gain, or obesity, is a much larger factor than drinking in reducing testosterone levels.

'If you drink excessively all the time,' he says, 'it increases the level of adipose fat, which puts up your body weight. This can get you into a horrible obesity spiral, where increased adipose tissue reduces your testosterone and also your muscles.'

The State University of New York conducted a study of 1,849 men over forty-five, which showed that obese people tended to have low testosterone levels, and that as the BMI increased, the testosterone levels went down. People with low testosterone values tended to put on more weight, and were more likely to develop diabetes. [29]

Which mean that the fatter you get, the less testosterone you have, the worse it gets, and the fatter you get. Oh, how scary is that ... ?

There's another thing you need to watch out for: the infamous nightcap.

'There's more research,' says Professor Horie, 'that shows that people get reduced testosterone values if they don't get much sleep. Alcohol has a stimulant effect, and lowers the quality of your sleep. And since it suppresses anti-diuretic hormones, as the effects wear off, you end up having to go to the loo several times during the night, which reduces your sleeping time still further.'

So, far from helping you get off to sleep, a nightcap can actually keep you awake and push down your testosterone levels! If you're in the habit of a drink before bedtime, you should watch out. Avoid drinking before bedtime, and get some good-quality sleep.

Reducing stress increases male hormones

Finally, is there a good way of drinking so you don't bring down your testosterone? I get that we should avoid drinking excessively,

---

29 Dhindsa, S. et al. 'Testosterone Concentrations in Diabetic and Nondiabetic Obese Men' in *Diabetes Care*; 2010, 33(6), 1186–1192.

and that beer on its own can have adverse effects, but how much is a reasonable amount? And *how* should we drink?

'As I said earlier, you don't need to worry if you don't drink excessively, because it has no direct effect on testosterone,' says Professor Horie. 'Just keep to the generally mandated 20g of pure alcohol, or one cup of saké a day, when you're drinking alcohol. If you try to swear off drinking completely, that will just be more stressful, and stress really *is* a major factor in diminishing testosterone! It is better for testosterone levels if you blow off steam and enjoy a moderate amount of alcohol. So I can recommend moderate drinking.'

However, I think the essential point, here, is when Professor Horie mentions that we should 'enjoy' it. Peer-pressure drinking, or intense man-to-man sessions can be stressful. The best thing is to enjoy drinking with people whose company you value.

'If you are in a male-only group, testosterone will be secreted. But if there is one or more women in the group, the secretion of testosterone increases even more.'

So an informal, relaxed drinking atmosphere is the best. Choose whom you drink with. But even if you are having fun, never drink to excess. [30]

Exercise increases testosterone levels

Additionally, you should really get into the exercise habit. Research exists that has confirmed that exercise stimulating the muscles will increase testosterone levels. [31] Apparently both aerobic workouts

---

[30] Translators' note – Japan's business culture often pushes company employees into compulsory work outings that are anything but fun. Some of the advice reflects such situations, particularly in such comments as 'choose whom you drink with'.

[31] Zmuda, J. et al. 'Exercise increases serum testosterone and sex hormone-binding globulin levels in older men' in *Metabolism*, 1996; 45(8): 935–9.

and muscular exercise are effective. To prevent testosterone-reducing obesity, exercise makes even more sense – so let's get on the move as often as possible without being lazy!

Get plenty of sleep, exercise, and enjoy drinking with people you like. Professor Horie's book *Hormone Ryoku ga Jinsei wo Kaeru* (*The Power of Hormones to Change Your Life*) suggests that the best way to increase testosterone levels is to be laid-back – live a comfortable life, laugh out loud, and reduce unnecessary stress. Keeping to a moderate amount of alcohol, you should release stress by laughing and drinking with your friends – that may well be the secret to delaying the decline of testosterone as you get older.

Periods, Pregnancy and the 'Pause – alcohol and women

Expert Adviser: Kazue Yoshino
Yoshino Women's Clinic

Oh, what in the world happened to my cast-iron liver?

As I get older, I get the feeling that I can't drink as much I used to. When I was in my twenties, I'd drink wine by the bottle, not the glass. If I went to a party, I would have a bottle of red, a bottle of white and a whisky chaser.

Back then, I was a writer for a weekly magazine, and I thought nothing about drinking until dawn, having a snooze, and then skipping out the door to the next interview. After my interviews were done, I'd go out on the town drinking until dawn again. And repeat. Back then, I had no idea what a hangover was, and even after drinking such a huge amount, my gamma-GTP was normal. I really was the owner of a cast-iron liver.

But once I hit my forties, if I drank a lot, I would suffer on the morning after. Then, as soon as I put one foot in the menopause, I entered an absolutely shambolic state of being unable to drink too much at all (although, come to think of it, I probably still put away a bit more than the average woman).

I'm not the only person this has happened to. Many women my age around me seem to complain that they can't drink as much as they used to. I've come to realise that although there are many different personal experiences, the menopause is a crucial time in forcing us to change our lifestyle, including the way we drink.

We already know that drinking can increase the risk of breast cancer for women (see p.135). The true causal relationship has yet to be understood, but we already know that the more you drink, the greater the risk. But are there any other risks from alcohol that women should be aware of? To start with, should women drink as much as men . . . ? I think I need to set the record straight.

So I asked Kazue Yoshino from the Yoshino Women's Clinic, a lady with an in-depth knowledge of menopausal disorders and female hormones.

Women have a lower alcohol tolerance!

For starters, do men and women have different levels of alcohol tolerance?

'Some women are large like me,' says Dr Yoshino, 'and every physique is different, but women tend to have livers that are smaller than men's. Women tend to be smaller, and have a lower alcohol tolerance. According to a report published by the National Hospital Organisation, Kurihama Medical and Addiction Center, women metabolise a lower amount of alcohol per hour, which makes their "alcohol metabolic rate" lower than men's.

'Also, we know that women have a smaller volume of blood circulation, which means that if a man and a woman both drink the same amount of alcohol, the woman, who is liable to be smaller, will have less blood to spread the alcohol around, so she will have a higher blood alcohol concentration. Alcohol stays in women's bodies for longer, which makes them more susceptible to its effects.

'Of course, our alcohol tolerance has a lot to do with our levels of alcohol metabolising enzymes, and *those* are determined by our genetic heritage. So there are some smaller women, like you, who seem to be able to hold a lot of drinks, so it differs from person to person, and it's impossible to say definitively that women are more lightweight drinkers. However, I think it's fair to say that there is a general tendency among women to be more susceptible to the influence of alcohol.'

I understand that even though there are variations in size or physique, women really shouldn't put booze away at the same pace as men, and they should try not to drink so much. There is no disputing that the amount our bodies can take is less than that of men.

According to Dr Yoshino, men and women show clear differences in the progress of alcoholic liver disease caused by drinking too much. Alcoholic liver disease is a scary affliction that can lead to cirrhosis if you carry on drinking to excess, but it affects women with greater speed than it affects men.

In fact, if you look up 'alcohol' in the Japanese Ministry of Health's twenty-first-century national health campaign, 'Healthy Japan 21', it clearly states that it is 'appropriate for women to drink less than men'. The same document's second target suggests that people are at risk of developing lifestyle diseases if they drink more than 40g of pure alcohol intake a day (for men) and 20g (for women). Surprisingly, the difference is double!

Because I am a heavyweight drinker, I paid no attention to this at all before, but women's physiques do generally make us more vulnerable to drink, and unable to manage the same pace as men. And 20g, as we should all know by now, is an amount of alcohol equivalent to one 500ml bottle of beer, two glasses (c.180ml) of wine or one cup of saké. I know it's a guideline, but it's such a tiny amount! Barely an aperitif for me . . . !

Periods, pregnancy and the menopause – three warnings

So, what do women need to worry about when they drink? Because of the menstrual period and ovulation, women's bodies have a huge variation in body condition and mental state. In addition, the menopausal period, which can take about a decade preceding and following the end of menstruation, also has a huge influence on women, physically and mentally. So, when should women be wary of drinking?

Dr Yoshino says there are three times when women need to watch their drinking: when they are pre-menstrual or menstrual, when they are pregnant, and during menopause.

'Currently, about 70 per cent of women suffer from some kind of pre-menstrual syndrome (PMS),' says Dr Yoshino. 'This means physical or mental discomfort, including bloating, excessive appetite and irritability, three to ten days before the menstrual period starts. We've yet to fully understand the causal relationship between PMS and female hormones like oestrogen and progesterone, but during this time, women can become depressed in addition to being in a poor physical condition. If you depend on alcohol to calm yourself down, you can end up with a habit and enter a vicious circle of constantly drinking more.'

Many women reading this are already nodding to themselves. I take an oral contraceptive to be free from PMS, but I used to suffer from it quite severely. I got aggressive rather than depressed when I got irritable, and when I drank, it got worse.

'Alcohol can only give you a moment's relief from a poor mental state,' says Dr Yoshino. 'It's more constructive to think about treating the root causes of PMS instead of drinking to take your mind off it.'

So what should we look out for when we are on our period?

'Women are influenced by prostaglandin, which is a kind of hormone that effects various elements of menstruation. Prostaglandin is a vital substance that contracts the uterus and pumps the menstrual blood, but at the same time, it can induce abdominal pains, headaches and nausea. Therefore, women are prone to nausea and headaches even without alcohol during their menstrual period. Drinking alcohol exacerbates that, which can cause drinking to make you feel even worse.

'Also, alcohol accelerates blood circulation and raises your pulse, increasing the amount of bleeding, which can cause anaemia. I think few women would choose to drink an excessive amount of alcohol during their period, but it's really a time when you should be drinking less.'

It varies from person to person, but I have heard people say that you can get sick-drunk when you are on your period. It seems smarter to stay away from the booze, and keep it to just a glass in company.

Three times for women to avoid drinking

menstruation	pre-menstruation	Avoid drinking alcohol to distract from discomfort caused by PMS (premenstrual syndrome).
	during menstruation	Alcohol exasperates the symptoms you get during menstruation. Avoid excessive drinking.
pregnancy		Never drink during pregnancy. It can harm the baby.
menopausal period		It is dangerous to rely on alcohol to distract from mental discomfort. Choose low-carb drinks, as a lowered metabolism accentuates weight gain.

Never drink when you are pregnant!

Women undergo physical and mental changes each month, but they also face some changes in the greater scheme of things. One of these changes is pregnancy, and as everybody ought to know already, never drink when you are pregnant. It's not like there aren't warnings on the side of alcoholic products.

'Alcohol has a huge effect,' says Dr Yoshino, 'not only on the pregnant woman, but also on her foetus. If the foetus develops Foetal Alcohol Syndrome (FAS), the baby can be born underweight or with brain damage that can affect it for life. You should avoid drinking during pregnancy.'

Menopausal women and alcohol dependency

But it's the aforementioned menopause that manifests itself as a truly huge mental and physical change sometime after women hit their forties. During this period, the sharp decline in oestrogen causes various physical disorders. One symptom is 'hot flushes', a sudden redness and hotness in the face, which can come accompanied by sudden sweating. The reduced output of oestrogen unbalances the autonomic nervous system, which controls the dilation of blood vessels. Many women suffer from this condition, and in some cases it can cause them to become withdrawn or depressed.

'The mental state is destabilised during menopause,' warns Dr Yoshino, 'so it's easy to reach for a bottle. Quite a few women develop alcohol dependency because of continual drinking during menopause.

'No good can come of depending on alcohol during this period. Even if you feel better when you are drinking, the anxieties will only come back when you sober up. To forget about them, you end up drinking again, and then you have to keep upping the amount of alcohol. Eventually, it's a road straight to alcoholism.'

Of course, this doesn't mean that you should give up drink altogether just because you are going through menopause. There's nothing wrong with enjoying a drink every now and then. But it is dangerous to rely on drinking as a crutch to cover an unstable mental state.

Women going through menopause suffer all kinds of bad conditions, such as sleep disorders and osteoporosis, as well as depression. We need to be particularly careful about insomnia. Many people drink to get off to sleep, which can become a habit and turn into a dependency on alcohol.

'Don't try to use alcohol to make up sleep,' advises Dr Yoshino. 'Try something else, like steering clear of caffeinated drinks later in the day, or stretching before going to bed. If you still cannot get to sleep, consult your doctor and consider sleeping pills.'

Choose low-carb drinks during menopause

While we're on the subject of menopause, there is something else to bear in mind, and that's obesity caused by a declining metabolism. I'm going through menopause right now, and find that unlike in my younger days, I put on weight really easily. If I'm not careful, I can put on five kilos without even trying.

'It's easy to gain weight, and difficult to lose it during your menopause,' says Dr Yoshino.

I know this to be true from personal experience, but still I can't stop drinking. What should I do . . . ?

'Your metabolism gradually declines from your twenties onwards,' she says. 'It should come as no surprise that you gain weight if you eat and drink the same quantities as you did when you were younger. I know women in my circle that put on ten or twenty kilos when they went through menopause. Some put on so much that it changed the shape of their faces, and I had trouble recognising them. So yes, you're going to put on weight during the period.

'All of which means you should choose your drinks carefully. From the point of view of avoiding weight gain, it's better to choose spirits like authentic *shōchū* and whisky without sugar. Brewed drinks, like beer and saké, contain more carbohydrates, although wine has a relatively low sugar content, so is a bit better than the others.'

'You should also try to avoid high-calorie, deep-fried foods and carbs in the bar snacks, like Japanese savoury pancakes and fried noodles. Instead choose low-calorie food like tofu or blanched vegetables in a *dashi* sauce.'

It gives me the shivers hearing I might put on ten kilos. But as Dr Yoshino points out, it's only natural that an older woman would put on weight if she kept drinking in the way she did when she was in her twenties. Regular exercise is a good way of avoiding menopausal weight gain – it's essential to bolster your declining metabolism with a little extra exercise.

Women's physical and mental condition can change dramatically every month, as well as over our lifetimes. Meanwhile, as society gets more egalitarian, we are getting more chances to drink alcohol with our colleagues . . . something we might want to review, along with how and what we drink.

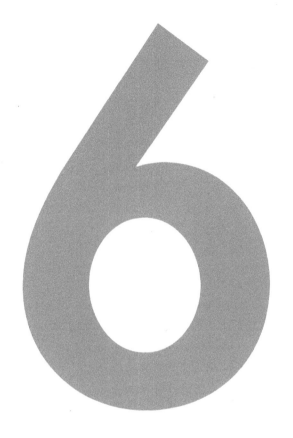

Drink and Be Merry – the healing power of alcohol

Smell the Roses – can shōchū fight off a blood clot!?

Expert Adviser: Hiroyuki Sumi
Professor emeritus, Kurashiki University of
Science and the Arts

Lifestyle illnesses like blood pressure and dyslipidaemia are a constant concern for the habitual drinker. Alcohol is said to increase your triglycerides, and has an effect on raising blood pressure. As we get older, our blood vessels age along with us and our blood changes, too. We can end up with something called 'thick blood', which is caused by a diet heavy in fats and carbs, a lack of regular exercise, and excess stress. It's not just about the booze – the extra calories from snacks while drinking are also a danger.

Eventually, thick blood can damage the endothelial cells of the blood vessels, creating a lump of blood – a blood clot. We can remain unaware while a blood clot gradually gets bigger in the blood stream, slowing down the blood flow or stopping it altogether to create serious, fatal conditions like arteriosclerosis, heart attacks or strokes. Blood clots are troublesome because they can pop up anywhere – in your arteries, your veins, your lungs, your heart or even inside the brain.

But there's good news for drinkers, because alcohol can be used to reduce the blasted blood clots. I asked Hiroyuki Sumi, Professor emeritus at Kurashiki University of Science and the Arts, about the blood-clot dissolving power of alcohol.

Certain shōchū drinks can double your blood thinning powers
'Blood clots are clumps of platelets within the bloodstream,' explains Professor Sumi, 'and they accumulate a fibrous protein called fibrin to become firmer "lumps" of blood. In a heathy body, the endothelial cells secrete enzymes that prevent blood clots, including substances like t-PA (the tissue Plasminogen Activator) and urokinase. These active an enzyme called plasminogen, which creates a proteolytic enzyme called active plasmin, and that breaks down fibrin and dissolves blood clots.

'But here's the thing – there have been experiments that reveal some alcohols have the power to accelerate t-PA and urokinase secretion. If you compare people who don't drink, with people who drink authentic *shōchū*, the drinkers' levels are actually almost double.'

How blood clots dissolve

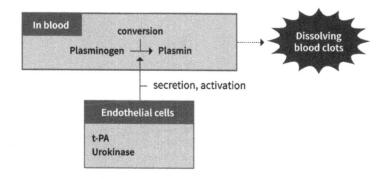

Substances secreted from endothelial cells, such as t-PA and urokinase, influence the plasminogen in blood plasma, which is a precursor to plasmin, the protein breakdown enzyme. Plasmin dissolves fibrin before it forms blood clots.

The spirit he mentions here is not multiple-distilled Kōrui or Ko-Otsu mix *shōchū* but a traditional *honkaku* (authentic) *shōchū* – a Japanese distilled alcohol, with an alcohol content less than 45 per cent and more usually about 25 per cent. There are various kinds of authentic *shōchū*, made from rice, wheat, barley and other ingredients, but Professor Sumi particularly recommends *shōchū* made from sweet potatoes (*imo-jōshū*), or Awamori, which is a rice-based liquor from Okinawa.

Shōchū and Awamori accelerate activity of t-PA

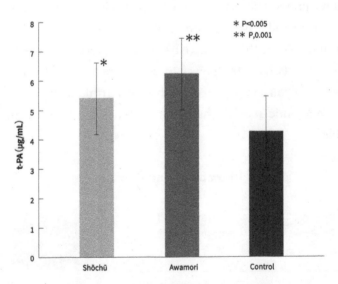

The study asked control subjects (twenty-four people), adults from the general public, to drink Awamori (fifteen people) or shōchū (nineteen people) and measured their subsequent t-PA activity. The results suggested that compared to the control group, the t-PA of both the shōchū and Awamori groups increased significantly. (Hiroyuki Sumi, "Functional Aroma Components in Shōchū: t-PA (Tissue Plasminogen Activator) Release and Platelet Aggregation Activity" in *Journal of the Brewing Society of Japan*, Volume 109, Issue 3, 2014, 137-146.)

'We tested twenty-four different kinds of *shōchū*, and discovered that certain sweet-potato varieties and Awamori increased the secretion and activation of t-PA and urokinase. Unfortunately, we haven't worked out yet just what it is in those brands that accelerates the activity of those two substances. We still don't know in detail how the mechanism really works for producing and secreting t-PA and urokinase. However, we have determined that the optimum amount for this effect is to take about 30ml in pure alcohol conversion per day.'

That is about 120ml of authentic *shōchū* – a piddling little amount that the average drinker is going to regard as a cruel torment. But by now we should all be aware that a moderate amount is going to be the best answer to anything.

'For the best health effects,' says Professor Sumi, 'it's best to drink just a little, and feel just a little tipsy.' And even though some *shōchū* brands are good for you in small doses, drinking them excessively will not multiply the anti-clotting effect any further.

Aroma alone can accelerate secretion!

It turns out that Professor Sumi's experiments did not merely prove that drinking certain types of *shōchū* have an effect. Even just smelling it can increase t-PA activity. [32] The secret lies somewhere in the unique flavour components of *imo-jōchū* and Awamori.

'There are many flavour components in *imo-jōchū*,' explains Professor Sumi, 'including beta-phenylethyl alcohol, one of the main fragrance components in roses, and ethyl caproate, which smells like apples. We found that the beta-phenylethyl alcohol was significantly powerful in activating t-PA. In other words, we can

---

32 Sumi, H. 'Shōchū no kaori seibun ga yūsuru shinki kinō-sei: t-PA (soshiki plasminogen activator) no hōshutsu, narabini kesshōban gyōshū yokusei kōka' [Novel functionality of shōchū scent components: release of t-PA (tissue plasminogen activators) and inhibitory effect on platelet aggregation] in *Jōkyō [Bulletin of the Brewing Society of Japan]* 2014; 109(3): 137–146.

expect a positive effect on dissolving blood clots even by simply smelling *imo-jōchū.*'

To be sure, there are quite a few people who find the smell of all those traditional ingredients in *imo-jōchū* to be relaxing. And if even smelling it has a positive effect, that's good news for those people who can't simply drink it.

Authentic shōchū has benefits for good cholesterol

So far, there has yet to be any comparable testing on other types of alcoholic drinks, but Professor Sumi has a theory.

'I have a hypothesis,' he says, 'that the secretion and the activation are caused by the relaxant effects of the aroma. So that should mean that it's not just *imo-jōchū* and Awamori, but other drinks, like brandy, which is loaded with flavour components, and fragrant forms of saké all might have a similar effect on the secretion and activation of t-PA and urokinase.'

Professor Sumi adds that authentic *shōchū* is good to drink and good to smell, but that it also has an additional health benefit.

'Authentic *shōchū*, along with *imo-jōchū* and Awamori, also has the effect of increasing "good cholesterol", or HDL.' HDL clears cholesterol off the vascular walls and carries it off to the liver, thereby reducing the risks of heart attacks or arteriosclerosis. Moreover, authentic *shōchū* contains no carbohydrates, and what could be better for drinkers who are worried about weight gain?

A new generation of young brewers has started pushing authentic *shōchū* and Awamori, recognising them for their taste and individuality. But let's not forget about their great health benefits, too!

Counter blood clots by eating
nattō with shōchū

Back on page 12, we discussed the value of *nattō* in combating hangovers. But it turns out that eating *nattō* while drinking *shōchū* has the additional benefit of being even better for dissolving blood clots.

'The stickiness of *nattō* comes from an enzyme called nattokinase, which breaks down proteins,' explains Professor Sumi. 'If you drink authentic *shōchū* and eat *nattō* alongside it, there's a synergy effect for dissolving blood clots. *Nattō* is often served with leeks, which also prevent blood platelets clumping in the first place, so it's all good for you.'

It was Professor Sumi himself who uncovered the health component in nattokinase. Tonight *nattō + shōchū* is going to be my new motto!

Red, Red Wine – why it's good for you

Expert Adviser: Michikatsu Satō
Institute of Enology and Viticulture,
Yamanashi University Graduate School

These days, wine is an entirely everyday drink in Japan. There have been more wine bars opening in recent years, and the *Izakaya* traditional bars, which used to offer beers and traditional Japanese drinks, have more wines in their selections. Thanks mainly to wines from the New World, like Chile and Australia, it has become easier for people to enjoy high-quality wines for less of a price.

The availability of wines at convenience stores and supermarkets has also plainly improved. Wine is no longer an expensive drink for important occasions, but has become something that you can enjoy every day. In fact, we are currently in the middle of Japan's seventh wine boom, and domestic consumption of wine is at its highest level ever.

And in the background of all this boom-time excitement, Japanese domestic wines are improving. Some have even won awards at international wine competitions like France's *Citadelles du Vin*.

Low French heart disease stats kicked off the boom

Japan went through a massive red-wine boom around the turn of the twenty-first century, after the media started highlighting the health benefits of red wine. Wine's rocketing popularity in Japan all boiled down to something called the French paradox.

The French paradox is based on the idea that French people have low rates of coronary heart disease, even though many of them are smokers, and their diet is rich in animal fats like butter and meat. It was the researchers Renaud and de Lorgeril who first began investigating the relationship between the consumption of dairy fats and wine in 100,000 French people, and comparing their rates of ischemic heart disease (heart attacks and angina).[33] Wine sales had been stagnating in America, but suddenly shot up again after CBS picked up the story. Over in Japan, the media similarly started discussing the benefits of red wine around 1997. People who had previously stuck to saké or *shōchū* suddenly gave wine a try instead.

With so much media attention, I am sure that you don't have to be a hard-core drinker to have already heard that the polyphenols contained in red wine are good for you. But you can get polyphenol from tea, as well – why aren't people talking about that? And why not white wine, or other alcoholic drinks? There are many questions flying around in my head.

So I put them all to Michikatsu Satō, a researcher in wine and polyphenol, now at the Institute of Enology and Viticulture, Yamanashi University Graduate School after working previously at the Mercian Corporation's Laboratory of Enology and Viticulture, Wine & Spirits Research.

To start with, what are polyphenols?

'It was the polyphenols that focused people's attentions on red wine,' says Dr Satō, 'because it contains a rich amount. Certainly,

---

33 Renaud, S. and de Lorgeril, M. 'Wine, alcohol, platelets and the French paradox for coronary heart disease' in *Lancet* 1992; Jun 20; 339 (8808): 1523–1526.

you can find polyphenols in tea and other beverages, including beers and saké, but the amount in red wine is overwhelmingly large. Compared to green tea, for example, red wine has six times as many polyphenols.'

Polyphenols always seem to come up when people are talking about the health benefits of wine, but what exactly are they?

'Polyphenols are components that make the colour and bitterness of wine, generated by photosynthesis. Polyphenols are made by large multiples of "phenol" units, which are structures comprising benzene rings shaped like tortoiseshells, with hydroxyl groups (OH) attached. The more OHs there are, the stronger the antioxidant effect. Which is to say, they protect our bodies from being damaged by active oxygen. They are chemical compounds generated by plants to protect themselves, so essentially you can find them in any plant. There are more than five thousand kinds of polyphenol, but the main ones to be found in red wine are anthocyanin, resveratrol and tannin.'

Polyphenol Structures

Phenol

An example of polyphenols
(the structure of resveratrol)

Polyphenols are multiple compounds of phenols (the one on the left). The more OHs there are, the stronger the antioxidative effect.

'But wine isn't merely rich in polyphenols; it also makes it easier for them to be absorbed into the human body. You'll find large amounts of polyphenols in fruits and vegetables, but in those forms, they are insoluble, and difficult for the human intestine to absorb. But in wine, they are present in a water-soluble state, so the body can absorb them more easily. There are a lot of polyphenols in the skin of grapes.'

Aha! And when you make red wine, you use the whole skin, juice and seeds of the grape. You leave it all to ferment, and even when the fermentation is done, you leave all the bits there for a while to soak, because that's what generates the unique colour and astringency. White wine, on the other hand, is fermented without the grape seeds or skins, which drastically reduces the polyphenol content.

Polyphenol content in the skins and seeds of grapes

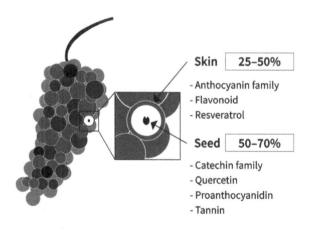

Skin 25–50%
- Anthocyanin family
- Flavonoid
- Resveratrol

Seed 50–70%
- Catechin family
- Quercetin
- Proanthocyanidin
- Tannin

Most of the polyphenols in grapes can be found in the skins and seeds. Grape juice contains some, but only a few per cent of the overall content.

Dr Satō says that there are even more polyphenols in wine that has been stored in a wooden barrel, because the polyphenol from the barrel wood will also seep into the wine. Wines with a strong wood aroma, even white wines such as many Californian brands, are also polyphenol-rich.

Cabernet has the best health effect!?

Let's take a closer look at the health benefits of red wine. There are several benefits from polyphenols, but the major one is their effect against ischemic heart disease and arteriosclerosis, as noted by Renaud and de Lorgeril. After their report was published, it inspired a series of follow-up studies examining wine's relationship to heart disease and arteriosclerosis.

'Dr Frankel from the University of California, Davis, compared polyphenols' antioxidant capabilities versus "bad" cholesterol (LDL) with vitamin E.[34] The results showed the polyphenols in red wine prevented LDL oxidation with half the concentration of vitamin E. This antioxidant effect is the important part. LDL cholesterol isn't bad in and of itself, but when it is oxidised by active oxygen, it causes arteriosclerosis. The polyphenols in red wine are effective in getting rid of the active oxygen. And my own experiments confirmed that anthocyanin (which is responsible for the colour of red wine) is a polyphenol that is highly effective at the removal of active oxygen.'

That has to be good news for drinkers with high cholesterol.

Dr Satō has also investigated the effects that the age of a wine has on its antioxidant effects.

'We were able to confirm that *mature* red wine has a greater antioxidant effect than younger wines. It reaches a peak after about five years, and after that, the effect gradually declines.'

---

34 Frankel, E.N. et al. 'Principal Phenolic Phytochemicals in Selected California Wines and Their Antioxidant Activity in Inhibiting Oxidation of Human Low-Density Lipoproteins' in *Journal of Agricultural and Food Chemistry*, January 1995, 43(4): 890–894.

As for the variety of grapes, Cabernet Sauvignon contains the most polyphenols and has the highest antioxidant effect. Cabernet Sauvignon is the variety used for Medoc in Bordeaux, Chile and many California wines, and it has a full body. In other words, full-bodied wine is better for your health.

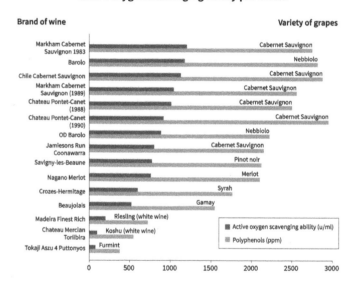

Difference in polyphenol content and active oxygen scavenging ability per brand

Active oxygen scavenging ability is the actual ability to eliminate active oxygen. The higher its value, the higher the antioxidant capability. Aged wine has stronger active oxygen scavenging ability. As for the variety of grape, Cabernet Sauvignon has proved to contain the largest amount of polyphenols. White wine also contains polyphenol, but the amount is smaller than that of red wine. (From publications by Professor Satō et al. in 1995-1996.)

Red wine is effective against dementia

On top of the antioxidant effects, the resveratrol also contained in grape skin is now attracting lots of scientific attention. This lesser-known polyphenol is said to facilitate brain functions, memory recovery and prevent Alzheimer's disease.

Correlation of wine consumption with dementia and Alzheimer's

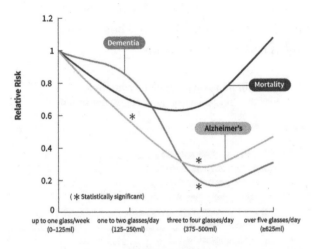

Amount of wine intake

These results are from a Centre Hospitalier Universitaire de Bordeaux study on 3777 people over sixty-five years of age for three years. Adapted from data received by Professor Satō from J. M. Orgogozo, one of the authors. (Orgogozo J.M., Dartigues J.F., Lafont S., et al., 'Wine consumption and dementia in the elderly: a prospective community study in the Bordeaux area' *Revue Neurologique*, Volume 153, Issue 3, 1997, 185-192).

'The Centre Hospitalier Universitaire de Bordeaux studied 3,777 people over sixty-five for three years,' explains Dr Satō, referring to a 1997 report. 'They checked their drinking levels and their mortality, along with the onset risks of dementia and Alzheimer's, and they found some amazing results. They compared a group in which the subjects drank three to four glasses of wine a day (375–500ml), and a group that did not drink wine at all. They found that the onset risk of dementia for the drinkers was a fifth of that for the teetotallers; it was a quarter for Alzheimer's, and the general mortality rate was 30 per cent less. This was believed to have been the result of resveratrol activating MAP kinase, an enzyme that responds to external stimuli.'

There was even a report that resveratrol activated Sirtuin, which has a function in suppressing ageing and prolonging people's lives. A paper published in 2006 suggested that resveratrol had been seen to prolong life in mice.[35]

The mice were reared on a high-calorie diet that should have shortened their lives, but those who were also fed resveratrol lived just as long as mice on a standard diet. The findings led pharmacies in the USA to sell out of resveratrol supplements. Japan, too, saw numerous manufacturers peddling supplements that purported to have 'anti-ageing' properties and 'activate long-life DNA'.

But a litre of red wine contains a whopping 10mg of resveratrol. So if you change your daily drink to red wine, you may find you enjoy the health benefits.

Red wine also has a bactericidal effect against helicobacter pylori. Test results from California State University, Fresno showed that off-the-shelf red wine impeded the proliferation of helicobacter pylori within 15 minutes (published in 1996). Dr Satō's own research, published in 1999, showed that it increased the flexibility of blood vessels, and the blood flow in the capillaries.

Looking at all these research results, it is understandable why red wine, among all the alcoholic drinks, gets so much attention.

Two glasses of wine is the appropriate amount for men

Having said that, if you drink too much, the harms outweigh the benefits. So what is a moderate amount?

'The range of what we call a moderate amount is from 10g to 30g a day in pure alcohol conversion. So that would be 100ml to 300ml, or roughly two glasses of wine. For women, the ideal

---

35 Baur, J.A, et al. 'Resveratrol improves health and survival of mice on a high-calorie diet' in *Nature* (2006) 444, 337–342.

amount would be at the lower end, around 100ml, because they are more susceptible to other risks from alcohol, such as breast cancer.'

But for a habitual drinker, two glasses of wine will never be enough.

'Two people could share a bottle between them,' suggests Dr Satō, 'which would be an acceptable level as long as they don't do it every day.' In other words, an amount we've heard elsewhere – about 150mg per week, assuming two liver resting days.

But even if you don't like red wine, you can still get the polyphenols out of it another way.

'The polyphenols in red wine are not easily destroyed by heat,' says Dr Satō. 'Even if you heat it up, about 60 per cent of them are left. So if you use it in cooking, it will make for a profoundly tasty dish, so it's kind of killing two birds with one stone.'

So, a glass of full-bodied red wine with a succulent beef bourguignon . . . which also has red wine in it. Just thinking about it makes my mouth water. It might be so tasty, however, that you end up drinking too much, and that will just lead to a hangover and cancel out all the health benefits. Remember, it is essential to do everything in moderation.

The Geisha's Secret – a skin lotion that gets you drunk

Expert Adviser: Saeko Wakazuki
Fukumitsuya

There was an old advert for luxury cosmetics which noted that the brewers and workers at saké breweries tended to have smooth, porcelain-like skin. It's been twenty years since I started working in the saké industry, but my skin condition is better now than it was in my twenties. I went to a cosmetics counter and asked them to check my 'skin age', and they told me that my skin is like that of a woman ten years younger than I actually am. I drink saké almost every day and use cosmetics made of saké. When I looked at the results, I thought: 'This must be the effect of all that saké.'

Similarly, it reminded me of an old lady I knew when I was a child. The town where I spent my early years before the middle of primary school used to be a fortress town, and many of the old ladies there used to be geisha. 'Granny at the tobacconist,' as we used to call her, was well over eighty years old but still had beautiful porcelain skin like a doll.

I told her how much I admired her skin, and she replied: 'When I was a geisha, if the clients didn't finish off their saké, I used to rub it into my face and neck.' Back then, I was still way too young to drink, but even forty years later, I still remember her beautiful skin, and her story that it was all down to saké.

I've noticed more and more beauty products with components of saké coming onto the market. Asahi Shuzo Saké Brewing in Yamaguchi Prefecture, the maker of the famous 'Dassai', is selling 'hand-made saké lees soap', and beauty conscious women have long favoured cosmetics using 'αGG', the saké-derived component developed by Hakushika (Tatsuuma-Honke Brewing Co., Ltd. in Hyōgo Prefecture).

Is it true that saké is good for your skin? Is it effective to apply saké on the skin? Which component of saké is effective? Many questions are brewing in my mind.

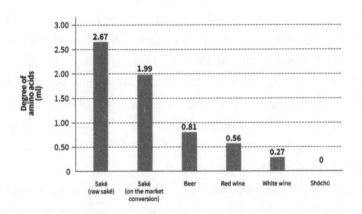

Amino acid content comparison of saké, wine, beer, etc.

Saké has a larger amino acid content compared with other alcoholic drinks. The data for this graph was based on an analysis by Fukumitsuya, using the company's own-brand saké. Other brands may vary in exact content.

I decided to put them to Saeko Wakazuki, who works as the store operations department manager at Fukumitsuya, a brewery in Kanazawa that was established in 1625. Fukumitsuya is an advanced brewery, which insisted on brewing saké only with rice during the time it was more usual to doctor it with extra alcohol. They have their own saké research centre, and are known to be also passionate about cutting-edge projects, as they started study into beauty products using rice fermenting technology in the 1990s.

Saké is overwhelmingly rich in amino acids!

'Saké contains many well-balanced varieties of amino acid,' explains Ms Wakazuki, 'including glutamic acid, alanine, leucine and arginine. Saké's amino acid content is about ten times more than that of white wine, by far the most in all the alcoholic drinks. Amino acids are an important component in proteins like collagen, which make up your skin. The main component of natural moisturising factor (NMF) found in the outermost layer of your skin is also an amino acid. Amino acids are essential substances for the skin, and we can call them "the foundation of beautiful skin". This is the reason why your skin feels supple when you put saké on your face.'

There are more than twenty kinds of amino acids in saké. From the viewpoint of moisturising, the most important one is serine. This is the main component of your own skin's natural moisturiser.

Apart from serine, saké contains other amino acids with natural moisturising factors, such as glycine, alanine, threonine and aspartic acid. So saké's skin-beautifying effect is not a myth! Let's not only drink saké, but, if there is any left, put that on our hands and face!

However, *junmai-shu*, which is for drinking, will be sure to moisturise your skin, but might be too stimulating for people with delicate skins or who cannot drink very much. Ms Wakazuki recommends 'putting a little bit on the skin of your inner arm, just to test beforehand that there will not be a problem'. If it is too strong for you, it is better to burn off the alcohol before you put it on your skin. But you will need to keep it in the fridge and use it within a week, as it does not contain any preservatives.

Major amino acids found in saké

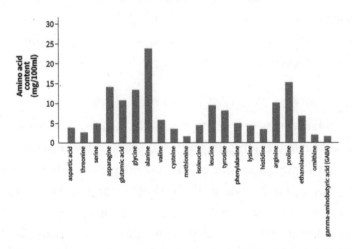

Saké is rich in more than twenty kinds of amino acid. The saké used for this sample was a *junmaishu* brewed by Fukumitusya. (Industrial Research Institute of Ishikawa).

Is junmai-shu better than junmai dai ginjō-shu?

But will just any old saké do? We mentioned earlier that are two types of saké. One has added brewer's alcohol (*honjōzō*). But fussy drinkers prefer the more basic kind (*junmai-shu*), which is saké made with nothing but rice, water and *koji*, the fermentation starter.

'It's *junmai-shu*, without the added alcohol, that is best for the skin,' says Ms Wakazuki. 'It has more amino acids.'

So, the traditional kind is the best, but will any *junmai-shu* do?

'Some people think that the more expensive variety, made with highly polished rice (*junmai dai ginjō-shu*) is best,' says Ms Wakazuki, 'but in fact, plain old *junmai-shu* is far better for the skin.'

That's good news for our pockets, at least, but why does the plain version have better cosmetic powers than the more expensive one? Apparently, it's to do with the way that the saké is made.

'The more polished the rice,' says Ms Wakazuki, 'the clearer and fruitier the taste of the saké. And *junmai dai ginjō-shu* is a prime example. But we reach that better flavour by reducing the amount of amino acids. If you're drinking it, a moderate amount of amino acids makes for a smoother taste, but if you're putting it on your skin, the more amino acids, the better. In other words, *junmai-shu*, because it has a harsher taste, is richer in amino acids and has a better effect on the skin.'

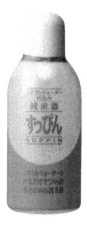

Fukumitsuya's Junmaishu Suppin, saké for applying on the skin. It is a proper saké with 13 per cent ABV. It is amino acid-rich. You can drink it, too.

How a Kanazawa geisha inspired a beauty product

Fukumitsuya has been researching cosmetics since the 1990s. There are more and more cosmetics with a saké component now, but how did they start developing them?

'The trigger came from a geisha in Kanazawa, in the district known as eastern Chaya-gai,' explains Ms Wakazuki. 'She was putting leftover saké on her face, and she had such wonderful porcelain skin. She said to me: "Saké is so good for your skin that you should really make cosmetics with it." On her recommendation, we developed a product called *junmai-shu suppin* – cosmetic saké. You're supposed to put it on your face, but if you really wanted to drink it, you could, because it is made just like standard *junmai-shu*.'

I was surprised that they came up with saké that was specifically for your skin. *Junmai-shu suppin* has a higher level of amino acids than normal saké, and the smell of alcohol disappears quickly because it is absorbed swiftly into the skin. However, its sales were hampered by the fact that even though it was supposed to be a cosmetic, it was technically an 'alcoholic drink' with a 13 per cent ABV. As a result, it could only be sold in liquor stores.

Fukumitsuya went back to the drawing board and spent several years developing Aminorice, an almost alcohol-free version, released in 2003.

Moisturising effects of rice fermentation liquid

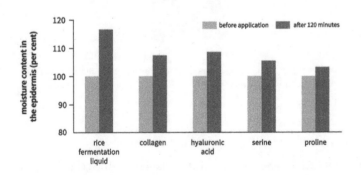

Comparison of moisture contents in the epidermis before and after application of the rice fermentation liquid used for *aminorice* on the skin for 120 minutes (research by Fukumitsuya). The rice fermentation liquid turned out to be more effective than collagen.

'The main ingredient in Aminorice is rice fermentation liquid,' says Ms Wakazuki. 'It takes forty days to take rice, *Aspergillus oryzae*, and yeast, with lactic acid bacteria, to make the rice fermentation liquid, and then we leave it to mature for more than six months. We let it go for that long because that ensures there will be a large amount of amino acids, better for the skin. It is fermented using a patented technology that prevents the creation of alcohol, but rest assured that the result is still a kind of saké, with a far heavier amino acid content than the saké you would usually drink.'

Aminorice contains a substantial amount of amino acids, including GABA, which improves the water content and prevents water loss in the upper layer of skin. It also has arginine, which keeps the skin layer flexible and moisturised to prevent chapped skin, and aspartic acid, which accelerates the skin's metabolism.

'The results we obtained showed a moisturising effect better than either collagen or hyaluronic acid,' she says. 'Also, it has a better antioxidant effect than vitamin C.'

When I put some on my skin, I hardly noticed any alcohol scent, and I could feel the skin becoming more supple almost as soon as I applied it. This is apparently because the molecules that make up amino acids are very tiny, a three-thousandth of the size of collagen molecules, allowing them to permeate deep into the skin. Never underestimate the power of an amino acid!

Thanks to the popularity of saké, Aminorice has many rivals today, also using saké ingredients as their inspiration. These include *Koji no Megumi*, produced by the Tsuchida Shuzō Brewery in Gunma Prefecture (where they make Homare Kokkō), *Daiginjō-shu Keshōsui Fukuchitose* from the Tajima Shuzō Brewery in Fukui Prefecture, made from rice fermentation liquid and saké lees, and *Komenuka Bijin* from Nihonsakari, which uses the rice bran created during the saké brewing process. It is difficult to choose between them.

Can you put saké in the bath?

If saké is good for the skin, can you have a bath in it? A well-known Japanese actress is said to like having saké baths, but do they actually have any effect?

'The alcohol component in saké can improve blood circulation, which can accelerate heat retention and perspiration,' says Ms Wakazuki. 'And the moisturising effects of the amino acids can make your skin smoother. On top of that, saké's unique aroma can have a relaxing effect. The appropriate amount of saké to put in your bath is about one or two cups.'

However, you must let the water out soonish, she warns, because the perspiration-inducing effect of alcohol will cause a lot of dirt to come out of your pores.

I tried saké in the bath once I had heard about it. I got sweaty sooner than usual, and after ten minutes or so, I felt dizzy. Judging from the line of dirt around the tub, there was certainly a detox effect. I used drinking saké in my bath, but you're probably better off with special 'bathing' saké. Products on the market include Fukumitsuya's *Suppin Sakéburō Senyō - Gen'eki*, which has a significant amino acid content, as well as *Sakéburo Nyūyoku Bijin* (from Chiyogiku), and *Yūyūbiteki* (from Suehiro Shuzo).

I'm sure the hard-core drinkers are already saying they would rather drink it than rub it in their face or pour it in their bath – see page 16 for the health benefits of drinking saké. But this saké beauty routine is sure to be popular with the ladies, so what have you got to lose?

Bitter Medicine – how beer can prevent dementia

Expert Adviser: Yasuhisa Ano
Kirin R&D Health Technology Laboratory

'Beer for starters.' [*Mazu wa beer!*]

You'll hear it all the time as you sit down at a Japanese style Izakaya bar. The drinker's best treat when they are parched is a cold beer straight down the hatch. But these days there are quite a few people who avoid beer, because it's a high-carb drink in a low-carb era. As far as I am concerned, if carbs are what's worrying you, you are better off watching the snacks you have with it than giving up on beer altogether.

And I would shout out from the rooftops: 'Beer is good for you!' Which is to say, beer can help prevent dementia.

Red wine is not the only dementia medicine

We've already discussed the role that the polyphenols in red wine can play in the prevention of Alzheimer's disease (see page 163), but research from the University of Tokyo, Gakushuin University and the Kirin brewery has revealed that the same effect can be found in beer. The research was published in November 2016 and widely reported in the Japanese media.

I'm getting on a bit now, and I increasingly find myself in embarrassing situations when I can't remember the names of people or things. I had a relative who developed dementia, so of course, I worry more often that I might end up suffering from it myself. So, naturally, when the news got out that beer could help, it suddenly grabbed the attention of me and every other drinker.

But is the story that beer has a protective effect against Alzheimer's really true? Beer is the most popular alcoholic drink, drunk by almost everybody. But unlike red wine, it hardly has the health-giving credentials that it might be actually good for you, particularly after we've already established that its carb-content brings a risk of weight gain.

And if it really is effective, does the same apply with low-alcohol flavoured beers or alcohol-free beers? So many questions in my mind, and who better to ask than one of the authors of the Kirin paper, Yasuhisa Ano from the Kirin R&D Health Technology Laboratory? He has been studying the health effects of beer for a long time.

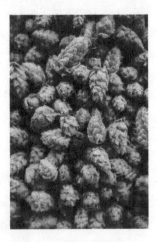

Hops, one of the ingredients used in beer, is an important element in imparting aroma and bitterness. It has been used as a medicinal herb since ancient times.

Beer-derived iso-α-acid clears up brain stains!

I got my answer right away.

'Beer contains what we call "iso-α-acid", which is a bittering component derived from hops,' says Dr Ano. The original 'α-acid' form is found in the resin gland of the hops flower, and when heated up in the brewing process, it turns into iso-α-acid and becomes effective. Without the brewing process, it doesn't work, so you can't get the same effect by just eating raw hops.

'Research has shown that iso-α-acid can prevent brain debris, such as amyloid beta peptides, from settling in the brain. This means it can reduce inflammation and improve cognitive function.'

So the thing that makes beer taste bitter will improve brain functions! Medicine can taste bitter after all . . . !

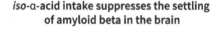

**_iso_-α-acid intake suppresses the settling
of amyloid beta in the brain**

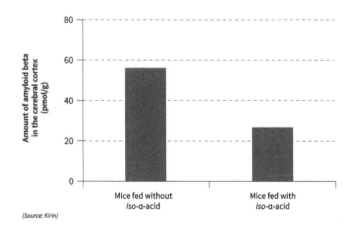

(Source: Kirin)

This requires a little explanation of exactly what Alzheimer's is. There are other types of dementia, including vascular dementia and dementia with Lewy bodies, but Alzheimer's is far and away the most common. It's said to be caused by malfunctioning brain neurons, which go wrong because of a build-up of proteins such as amyloid beta peptides in the brain.

For the experiment, the researchers used Alzheimer model mice – mice at the University of Tokyo that have been genetically modified to get Alzheimer-causing build-up early. The scientists put traces of iso-α-acid in the mice's food for three months. When the time was up, the mice who had been fed iso-α-acid showed a substantial suppression of brain detritus, compared to a control group of mice who had just been fed normally. In fact, they had half as much.

iso-α-acid suppresses inflammation in the brain

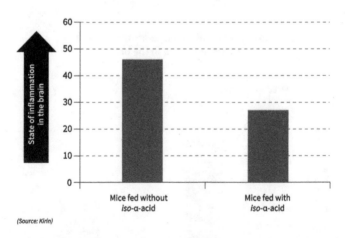

(Source: Kirin)

The vertical axis shows the amount of a physiologically active substance called cytokine, which is released when the brain is inflamed (unit is ug/g). The larger the value, the more inflammation there is in the brain. (Source: Kirin.)

'Particularly notable was the suppression in the hippocampus and the cerebral cortex, which is responsible for memory,' explained Dr Ano. 'Amyloid beta, as it were, is like a stain in the brain. This is thought to contribute to Alzheimer's, and once it builds up in the brain, the neurons responsible for cognitive function and memory don't work so well. We forget things, or get confused. Ageing is a root cause, but so is lack of sleep.'

So the test on mice confirmed that brain inflammation was reduced by 50 per cent. They carried out a behavioural evaluation of the mice, and confirmed that their memory retention was also improved.

Iso-α activates the brain's clean-up cells

So, how does this work? Dr Ano explains that the key lies in brain cells called microglia.

'The microglia are the only immune cells in the brain,' he says. 'We also call them the brain's clean-up cells, because they eat and remove debris like amyloid beta. They are important cells for repairing brain tissue, for the day-to-day development of synapses, and also protection from viruses.'

I never knew that there were such clever cells inside my brain. This all sounds really promising.

'However,' continues Dr Ano, 'as microglia function declines with age, the brain's ability to sweep away the amyloid beta deteriorates. They might overreact inside the brain, causing inflammation and generating active oxygen, which can damage the neurons nearby. But the iso-α-acid in hops can stimulate the microglia. It gets them active again, and the debris has more trouble settling, the inflammation goes down and Alzheimer's is prevented.'

Wow, let's hear it for beer. I am sorry now that I ever thought it would have fewer health properties than wine. It's still surprising to hear that beer has hidden effects.

'The hops in beer have been prized in traditional medicine for over a thousand years,' says Dr Ano. It was because of this long history that he focused on it as his research topic.

Beer improves the brain's communication function

That's all very well for the mice, but what about the effect on the human body?

In fact, before he even got going with the mice, Dr Ano had used fMRI (functional magnetic resonance imaging) to verify the effect of iso-α-acid on the human brain. In March 2016, he had already showed that ingestion would improve the brain's ability to process data and communicate. The study was adopted as a national ImPACT project by the Japanese Cabinet Office, and won the top prize.

'The participants in the study were twenty-five healthy people between the ages of fifty and seventy. We got them to drink 180ml of a non-alcoholic, beer-like drink that contained iso-α-acid every day for four weeks. Of that 180ml, the iso-α-acid content was 3mg. We took fMRI images before and after they drank and analysed the thickness of the cerebral cortex and that of nerve fibres. The test results suggested that a moderate intake would potentially improve the brain's communication function. We found that it was particularly effective on the over-sixties.'

You'll note that they used alcohol-free drinks in this experiment. As we already know from discussion of the J-Curve Effect (see page 65), there is already research suggesting that moderate alcohol intake might have a beneficial effect in preventing dementia. In order to exclude alcohol from skewing the results, and to show the pure effect of iso-α-acid alone, the researchers left alcohol out of the drink.

Which beer is good? How much should we drink?

If beer is good for you and can hold off Alzheimer's, what kind of beer is best, and how much should we drink? There's so much to choose from, with a thriving beer market including imported beers, sparkling ales, microbreweries and alcohol-free brands.

'A normal beer has about ten to thirty parts-per-million of iso-α-acid,' says Dr Ano. 'The bitter ones, like the IPAs, contain a little more. The non-alcoholic beer we used for the test had between twelve and thirty parts-per-million.'

Okay, so bitter is better. It's good news for the non-drinkers that the alcohol-free beers also have the same effect. But how much should we have?

'At this moment, all I can identify is a beneficial effect in preventing Alzheimer's. We haven't reached the stage yet where I could rule on an appropriate amount. But first of all, the most important thing is to keep within a moderate amount, to avoid undoing all the good work by causing yourself harm through excessive drinking. You can enjoy the effect of iso-α-acid even from non-alcoholic beer, so the elderly and people with low alcoholic tolerance do not need to force themselves to drink beer.'

This interviewer was kind of hoping to hear 'the more, the better', but sadly I am once again confronted with the word 'moderate'. You are probably sick of reading it by now, but a moderate amount means 20g in pure alcohol conversion for men, or a single 500ml bottle of beer or two glasses (c.180ml) of wine.

I'm sure some people would prefer to be told they should drink more, but even so, this has to feel like permission to crack open a beer, even for those who had started avoiding it. It's great for me, because now I have a new reason to enjoy a beer.

On top of that, iso-α-acid has other positive effects, including lifestyle illness prevention, weight loss, hypertension improvement, and suppression of greying hair. The prevention of lifestyle illnesses is particularly important, because they too can be causes of dementia. It is more stressful to resist your desire to drink. Now, let's say cheerfully: 'Beer for starters!'

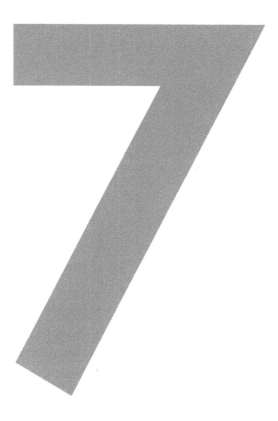

Drinking Dangerously –
things you must
never do

Wake-Up Call – nightcaps are only temporary and can cause depression

Expert Adviser: Miki Satō
Shimbashi Sleep Mental Clinic

Have you ever reached for a bottle to help you sleep, when anxiety or irritation are keeping you awake, or even because you are too excited? Thanks to the power of alcohol, your eyelids start to droop and you manage to fall asleep. Sure, we've all been there. But whether that actually amounts to a good night's sleep is another matter. Sometimes, I wake up just a few hours later, and my eyes are wide open after that. I am sure many people, not just the hard-core drinkers, have had some sort of similar experience.

Many people think that a nightcap will help get you off to a sound night's sleep, but is that really true? There's actually research data that confirms that 48.3 per cent of Japanese men (nearly one in two!), and 18.3 per cent of Japanese women have a nightcap at least once a week.[36]

I asked Miki Satō from the Shimbashi Sleep Mental Clinic, who has in-depth knowledge of the correlation between sleep and alcohol, and has a good track record of treating alcohol-related insomnia.

---

36 Kaneita, Y. et al. 'Use of alcohol and hypnotic medication as aids to sleep among the Japanese general population' in *Sleep Medicine* 2007, Nov(8), 723–732.

Alcohol deepens the first stage of sleep

'There are two kinds of sleep,' explains Dr Satō. 'Shallow REM (rapid-eye movement) sleep and deep (non-REM) sleep. There are also four depths of sleep, depending on the brainwaves and neuron activity. If you go to bed after drinking alcohol, we know that the time it takes you to fall asleep is shortened, and slow wave sleep, which is deep sleep in stages three and four, is increased. The longer and deeper you sleep, the more you secrete the growth hormones that are necessary for repairing your body cells.'

That sounds familiar – when I go to sleep after drinking, I fall asleep quickly and feel like I am in a deep sleep, which is apparently the thing that Dr Satō calls 'slow wave sleep'. So, on that basis, a hard-core drinker will happily take away the message that a nightcap can increase the quality of sleep. But they'd be wrong.

Sleep comprises REM sleep and non-REM sleep

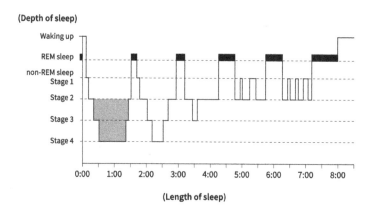

The deep sleep reached at Stage 3 and Stage 4 after falling asleep is called 'slow wave sleep' (the grey area of the above graph). Slow wave sleep accelerates the secretion of the growth hormones that repair cells and rest the brain.

Nightcap benefits wear off within a week

'If we look solely at the slow wave sleep after the first stage of sleeping,' says Dr Satō, 'a nightcap does seem to increase the quality of sleep. However, there's a rebound brought on by the alcohol, because the shallow sleep (REM sleep) lasts longer, and that's the period where you are more likely to wake up during the night. In other words, looking at the whole night, alcohol reduces the overall quality of your sleep.'

Then, what is causing the rebound that makes sleeping harder?

'It's the acetaldehyde that is produced when alcohol is broken down in the liver,' he explains. 'It increases in the blood stream and reaches the brain, where it impedes the brain's normal rest during sleep. Instead, it pushes up the sympathetic nervous system (SNS), otherwise known as the fight-or-flight response. That's what wakes you up.

'A nightcap will stop helping you sleep after three to seven days, so you end up drinking more to compensate, sometimes without even realising it. It ends up lowering the quality of your sleep still further and increasing the risk of alcohol dependency.

'Initially,' adds Dr Satō, 'alcohol gives you a sense of relaxation and happiness because of the GABA neurotransmitters in the brain, connecting, as they should, to $GABA_A$ receptors. At the same time, it inhibits Glutamate, an excitatory neurotransmitter, and NMDA receptors, which accelerates the process of falling asleep. You can quickly achieve a state of deep sleep. On the other hand, the $GABA_A$ receptors get used to it fast, causing you to increase the amount of alcohol, and heightening your dependency. Since the nightcap effect will be gone within a week at most, maybe you started off with a nightcap of 350ml of beer, but then the amount increased, to a 500ml bottle, and then a whole litre. This is why it's important to get out of the habit of needing a nightcap to get to sleep.'

Nightcap aid in falling asleep and increasing slow wave sleep

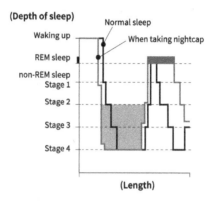

Alcohol helps us to fall asleep quicker and the time it takes to reach Stage 3 and Stage 4 is quicker, increasing the time of slow wave sleep. However, because of the rebound effect, REM sleep becomes longer, which is believed to cause nocturnal awakening. (The graph was created by the *Gooday* editorial team based on the interview.)

Nightcaps can cause sleep disorders and depression

According to Dr Satō, if you keep relying on alcohol to the extent that low-quality sleep becomes a chronic condition, your body activates a defence mechanism called hypervigilance – a state of constant physical and mental stress.

'So, to use a familiar example, if you work through the night without any sleep, you feel physically and mentally tired, but you can't get to sleep even after you have gone to bed. If you get into that situation, your sleep patterns are disrupted, and you become irritable. You snap easily, because your sympathetic nervous system is in a constantly heightened state, and in more serious cases, you will develop depression.'

The impact of a nightcap on the human body turns out to be far greater than I had imagined. But in that cast, how can we get good quality sleep back once we give up on the alcoholic crutch?

'Based on my experience of treating patients,' says Dr Satō, 'if your sleep pattern is so disrupted that you develop hypervigilance, even if you stop drinking alcohol, in some cases it can take up to six months to get back to a normal sleeping pattern.'

Check your 'sleep regime' before relying on a nightcap

The risk of sleep disorder persistently haunts us even after we stop taking a nightcap. The easiest way to get out of the nightcap habit is to stop keeping booze at home, but that sounds like too harsh an option for the habitual drinker. Isn't there a remedy that we can try without stress?

'I don't recommend using drinking as a means of getting to sleep,' says Dr Satō, 'but equally, if you keep to a moderate amount for meals or relaxing, that's not going to affect your sleep. If you do drink too much, it's better to flush yourself out by drinking water before bedtime, in order to lower your blood alcohol concentration. Based on these steps, and with a good sleep regime, the quality of your sleep should gradually improve.'

Sleep regime checklist by Dr Satō

- Have a bath (or a shower) at least two hours before going to bed
- Bathwater should not be too hot, make it c.40 degrees Centigrade
- Stop using smartphones and computers at least one hour before bed
- Do not go to brightly lit places, such as convenience stores, late at night
- Get up at the same time each morning, even at weekends

Dr Satō uses this sleep regime checklist with his patients, and it's a relatively simple set of steps that even a child could carry out, such as a regular bathtime, moderate water temperature, light control and a fixed wake-up time. It doesn't look difficult to manage.

If you still cannot avoid taking a nightcap . . .

If you still can't stay away from nightcaps, then you may have to try the last resort.

'We know from various research reports that chronic low sleep quality can raise your risk of developing a lifestyle illness, such as high blood pressure, diabetes or metabolic syndrome,' says Dr Satō. 'Also, alcohol acts as a muscle relaxant on the throat, narrowing the respiratory tract and causing sleep apnoea or aggravating snoring. If you're aware of these risks and still can't get to sleep without a nightcap, I recommend you visit your doctor for a prescription of sleeping pills. The Japanese tend to be afraid of sleeping pills, but speaking as a doctor, alcohol that can mess up the body in just a few hours is far scarier! These days, it's easier to get sleeping pills that aren't addictive, so it is worth considering them.'

Even if you think you got a good night's sleep thanks to a nightcap, it won't have been enough if your work performance is badly affected, or if you feel sleepy during the daytime. The best way to gain a good quality sleep is to be aware that while it's okay to enjoy alcohol, you should not use it as some sort of knock-out drug.

Read the Label – never mix drink and drugs

Expert Adviser: Hisashi Iijima
Chiba Pharmaceutical Association Drug Information Center

Drinkers can't leave their drinks alone, even when it turns chilly outside, and colds and flu are on the rampage. On the contrary, you'll hear them claim that they are disinfecting the virus with some alcohol, which is an excuse to drink even more than usual.

But no matter how much 'disinfecting' you think you are doing, you can never win forever against viruses. You're going to catch a cold eventually, and then you have no choice but to take medicine. But it's in the nature of the hard-core drinker that you want to drink even when you have to take medicine. I've done it myself, I've even gone out on the town after taking my medicine. Very occasionally, I will take it with beer . . .

But even I know that you should take medicine with plain water. In fact, every time I see my doctor to get medicine for something, I am told that I have to refrain from drinking alcohol, although I don't always follow the restrictions to the letter. I know . . . I just do it.

Luckily, I have never had any problems so far. There was a time when I took painkillers and cold remedies along with alcoholic drinks, which made me nauseous but didn't get me into a lot of trouble. I still take medicine before or after drinking.

So, what are the risks if you take medicine with alcohol? I asked Hisashi Iijima from the Chiba Pharmaceutical Association Drug Information Center about the correlation between drugs and booze.

As expected, mixing drink and drugs is a no-no

'Taking medicine with alcohol!?' he exclaims. 'Out of the question! Absolutely not. The golden rule is to take medicine with water.'

Well, that told me. I knew it all along, of course, but probably because I have never felt at serious risk, I have often ignored this advice. But what really is the problem?

'Alcohol affects the way that many medicines work, and the effect can be different from drug to drug. Typically, for example, it risks either enhancing the medicine's effects, or even its side effects. Alcohol and medicine, as many people may know, are both metabolised in the liver, and they are metabolised by the same enzyme, CYP2E1 (cytochrome P450). If they both hit the liver at the same time, they end up fighting over the enzyme.

'So let's say we've got a drug and 50 per cent of it is usually metabolised by the enzyme. If alcohol is halving the enzyme's effect, then only 25 per cent of it is metabolised, and the other 75 per cent of it gets into the blood stream. The medicine's dosage is based on the assumption that half of it will be metabolised, but because of this, we've delivered a dose that's half again as large as we planned. In pharmacological terms, it is working too effectively.'

Oh no, so alcohol makes medicine work *too* well. Certainly, that can't be good news for the body.

'On the other hand, if you consume alcohol every day, you have high enzyme activity. It can mean that you metabolise too much of the medicine, which means it is less effective.'

It can cause life-threatening critical conditions

Hmm, so it seems there really are risks for mixing drinks and drugs, including that the medicine can either become too strong, or not strong enough. But Dr Iijima hasn't finished with his examples.

'So, as an example of accelerated pharmacological effects, we use warfarin to treat blood clots. If ordinary people take warfarin with alcohol, it gets too strong and can cause haemorrhaging. If the haemorrhaging happens in the brain, it could be a life-threatening critical condition.

'But then again, there are medicines that can become too weak. The same dose of warfarin, if administered to a heavy drinker, might be processed too efficiently by their high enzyme activity, leaving little of it left to actually get to work. So you think that you are taking a drug to help you, but actually, your body is still susceptible to blood clots, and you have a greater risk of heart attack or stroke.

'But there's more. Because if you are taking metformin, which is used in the treatment of diabetes, an excessive alcohol intake will reduce your body's ability to process lactic acid (leading to lactic acidosis). Too much lactic acid can have an adverse effect on the central nervous and digestive tract, so extra caution is necessary.'

This is scary . . . ! It's bad enough being sick-drunk, but being sick-drunk while taking medication might even be hazardous to life. Having said that, the medicines Dr Iijima is talking about are prescription drugs. If you don't have thrombosis or diabetes, you might think the rules don't apply to you . . . right?

Caution is required even with cold medicine and painkillers

So, how about painkillers and cold medicines that we keep at home, easily available over the counter at a pharmacy?

'Well, of course,' says Dr Iijima, 'there are many over-the-counter medicines that require caution. Paracetamol, for example, which is a common ingredient in painkillers and cold remedies, is discharged from the body mainly through three metabolic pathways – glucuronic acid conjugation, sulfate conjugation and CYP2E1. CYP2E1 turns paracetamol to N-acetyl-P-benzoquinone imine (NAPQ1). This NAPQ1 is toxic to the liver, but when combined with glucuronic acid, it gets discharged as mercapturic acid. However, for habitual drinkers, induction of CYP2E1 accelerates the generation of NAPQ1 and exceeds the limit of glucuronic acid conjugation, which leads NAPQ1 to build up and cause a liver disorder.'

I see. As a habitual drinker, I need to be particularly careful . . . I regret it now, after all this time.

Hay now – what about allergic rhinitis?

Okay then, what about hay fever.

'Medicines for hay fever, or allergic rhinitis, used to come with warnings that they would make you drowsy if you took them with alcohol. These days, it is possible to get some medications that don't have quite such a knock-out effect on the central nervous system, such as Fexofenadine (product name: Allegra), so the situation is changing. However, the effects on the central nervous system vary from product to product. Please ensure you talk to an expert about any individual medicine.'

I use anti hay-fever drugs during the allergy season, and I've noticed I have been less drowsy than I used to be. However, it sounds like it would be smarter to stop taking them along with alcohol if the correlation between their effects isn't well known.

Wait three to four hours after drinking

These examples are only the tip of the iceberg. Although the effects can vary, I now totally understand that I should avoid taking medicine with alcohol. But there must be many hard-core drinkers who can't imagine a day without booze. If we have to take medicine three times a day, when will we be able to enjoy a drink? And what about people who take medicine to help their digestion before a party? What about them?

So, for starters, how long should we wait after drinking to take our medicine?

'Well, if you're taking medicine,' warns Dr Iijima, 'I'd really prefer it if you weren't drinking at all. The time alcohol takes to dissipate in the body varies, depending on someone's bodyweight and gender. The Health and Medicine of Alcohol Association says that it takes about three to four hours for one unit (20g of pure alcohol = 500ml bottle of beer or 1 cup of saké) to dissipate for an adult man weighing 60 kg.[37] This is only a rule of thumb, but wait for at least three to four hours.'

I see. So if we're taking medicine, we need to wait three or four hours for the alcohol to get out of its way. However, if the alcohol intake goes up to *two* units, then the alcohol stays in the body for six to seven hours, so you have to wait even longer.

So what about drinking after taking medicine? What about medicine taken to aid digestion?

'I can't put a number on how many hours you need to wait, because every medicine has its own rate of metabolising and rate of elimination. That said, it's fine to take medicine to protect or repair gastric mucosa, or a health drink to protect the liver, before drinking alcohol. However, there are some medicines that you just cannot combine with alcohol, so make sure to consult with an expert beforehand.'

I see. I am one of those people, but there must be many others, who take health drinks that are supposed to be good for the

---

37 For more details, check out the Health and Medicine of Alcohol Association website: http://www.arukenkyo.or.jp/health/base/ (in Japanese only)

digestive organs or the liver. Apparently, thank God, those are fine. But follow Dr Iijima's advice, and do check with your physician or pharmacist when buying medicine you plan to take at around the same time as drinking alcohol.

When you catch a cold, say no to alcohol and proclaim a liver holiday. After all, the best medicine for a cold is rest, so let your hard-working liver have one, too.

Smell You Later – watch out for bad breath

Expert Adviser: Tatsuo Yamamoto
Kanagawa Dental University

I'm sure plenty of drinkers out there have had a telling-off from their family about bad breath, when they've got home . . . or even by a colleague back at work the next day. Maybe they were too drunk to brush their teeth, or did a slapdash job before going to bed, but many hard-core drinkers have breath bad enough to turn heads. In fact, you can acquire a smell of alcohol, but what really matters to the people nearby is the strong, fishy, rotten smelly breath.

Is it alcohol that makes your breath smell so bad? I asked Tatsuo Yamamoto, a professor at the Department of Oral Science, Kanagawa Dental University Graduate School of Dentistry.

'Alcohol isn't the only cause of bad breath,' he says. 'In most cases, bad breath is caused by gum disease. We believe that anaerobic bacteria, generated by periodontal gum disease, propagate in the mouth, producing smelly gases like hydrogen sulphide and methyl mercaptan.'

Gum disease is a generic term for disease in the tissues surrounding the teeth.

'It's caused by oral bacteria and plaque, including that generated by the bacteria,' explains Professor Yamamoto. Plaque gets into periodontal pockets between the teeth and gums, causing inflammation and eventually dissolving the alveolar bone. It is, as it were, a hotbed for bacteria. If you ignore it, you might end up losing your precious teeth. According to research by the Japanese Ministry of Health, Labour and Welfare, the rate of gum disease in those aged between fifty-five and seventy-four is more than 50 per cent.[38]

Alcohol aggravates gum disease

But if bad breath is caused by gum disease, what causes the gum disease? Is alcohol anything to do with it?

'We don't yet clearly understand the mechanism by which alcohol might aggravate gum disease,' says Professor Yamamoto. 'However, there have been epidemiological studies that have demonstrated that people who drink more alcohol have a higher rate of gum disease.'

What!? So then alcohol and gum disease are not unrelated . . .

Research in Korea investigating 8,645 men of around forty years old, found that those who were habitual drinkers had a 1.27 times higher risk of gum disease than those who did not drink.[39] Similar research conducted on 1,115 people in Brazil showed that women who daily drank more than 9.6g of pure alcohol (about half a cup of saké) were at 3.8 times more risk of developing gum disease than those who did not drink.[40] Professor Yamamoto's own research, carried out on rats, has revealed a connection between alcohol and gum disease.

---

38 *Survey of Dental Diseases*, 2011.

39 Park, J. et al. 'Association Between Alcohol Consumption and Periodontal Disease: The 2008 to 2010 Korea National Health and Nutrition Examination Survey' in *Journal of Periodontology* 2014; 85: 1521–1528.

40 Susin, C. et al. 'The association between alcohol consumption and periodontitis in southern Brazilian adults' in *Journal of Periodontal Research* 2015; 50: 622–629.

'When we fed excessive alcohol – an amount that would have got a human drunk if scaled up – to rats without gum disease, the alveolar bone that supported the teeth was significantly degraded. We also found out that active oxygen was produced around the bone, and the body's antioxidant properties were lowered. On that basis, we can suggest that alcohol does not only heighten the risk of gum disease, but that the progression of gum disease can increase the body's risk to active oxygen.'

Professor Yamamoto goes on to point out that because alcohol suppresses the anti-diuretic hormone, making urine discharge more frequently, its hydration drops and this causes a decrease in the amount of saliva. This worsens the oral environment, and helps the bacteria propagate.

'And if you throw in smoking as well,' he adds, 'it just gets even worse.

'There is a report that says that the risk of gum disease for smokers is up to eight times higher than the risk for non-smokers. This is because smoking slows the blood circulation in the gums, and plaque can easily stick to tar, creating a powerful bacterial periodontal disease called biofilm.'

The bad breath caused by gum disease can end up rupturing human relationships. But what if, like me, it's impossible to give up drinking altogether? Is there anything we can do to prevent gum disease?

'There is no better way to ward off gum disease than brushing your teeth,' says Professor Yamamoto. 'There is no time that is particularly better for brushing, so it is important to take the time to brush your teeth properly in the morning, during the day and in the evening.'

Sluice twice to keep the effect

There's something I've been meaning to ask about brushing. I've heard some people say that it is better to avoid brushing your teeth for thirty minutes after eating. Is it better not to brush your teeth after drinking alcohol?

'To be precise,' says Professor Yamamoto, 'it's not thirty minutes after eating, but thirty minutes after eating acidic food. There have been reports in the West that people who drink a lot of wine can get acid erosion on the enamel on their teeth.'

What can wine lovers do to prevent acid erosion?

'If you want to actively prevent it, brush your teeth with a fluoride toothpaste before drinking. Fluoride has the effect of reducing the risk of acid erosion by promoting calcium intake (recalcification) from saliva and strengthening the quality of the teeth. By coating the teeth in advance with fluoride, you can expect to soften the impact of acidic drinks, including wine. Quite a few drinkers avoid doing it because they say that the toothpaste changes the taste of their drinks. Such people should brush their teeth about an hour before they start drinking.'

And there is a key to doubling the effect of fluoride.

'Try to only sluice a couple of times after brushing. If you rinse your mouth so much that the taste of the toothpaste has gone, then you have washed away all the fluoride that you applied. You might find that just sluicing once or twice isn't enough, particularly if you have a strong fluoride toothpaste, but once you get used to it, it becomes a habit.'

I tried to take his advice, and it did take some getting used to. After several days, I overcame my resistance. You can start a new habit tonight of brushing your teeth before you start to drink.

Fight off gum disease with the toothpick method!

Brushing is the key to preventing bad breath. But brushing teeth for the sake of it is not good enough. Professor Yamamoto came up with his toothpick method after years of research. The method requires nothing other than the toothbrush you are already using. Using this method, he said, gum disease can be prevented.

Prevent gum disease with gum massage

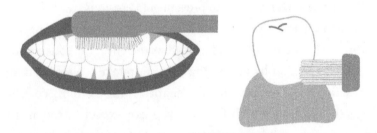

For the front of the front teeth, apply the tip of the brush at the borderline between the teeth and the gum and move the toothbrush towards the tip of the teeth. For the rear teeth, apply the brush at a right angle and vibrate the brush. For the backs of the teeth, use the tip of the brush and push it in and out in the gap between the teeth.

'Gum disease starts between the teeth,' he explains. 'The toothpick method massages the gum between the teeth and revives the crevicular epithelium, the contact between teeth and gums, which has become fragile. Apply the tip of the brush at the borderline between the teeth and the gums, downwards for upper teeth, and upwards for lower teeth, and brush up and down ten times in place. For the back of the teeth, use the tip of the brush and push it in and out in the gap between the teeth ten times for each place. The pressure should be just as much as when you use a rubber eraser on a letter. It takes about seven to eight minutes altogether, but it goes very quickly if you do it while watching television.'

In fact, Professor Yamamoto brushed my teeth using the toothpick method, and I felt the surface of my teeth became smooth and gums becoming firmer. It differs from person to person and depending on age, but Professor Yamamoto's research has revealed that if you keep using the toothpick method, gum disease can improve in one to six months.

Bad breath is difficult to spot by ourselves, and it is hard for the people around us to point it out, so treatment gets delayed. To prevent people holding their nose as soon as you open your mouth, please keep these cares in mind, and keep to drinking a moderate amount.

Heat Shock – the risks of drinking in a winter bath

Expert Adviser: Satoshi Umemura
Director of Yokohama Rosai Hospital

I bet I am not the only one who feels like a hot bath after a few drinks. Drunken drinkers can get bolder, and end up saying: 'Let's have a bath to sweat out the alcohol.' Except you can't actually 'sweat out' the alcohol.

In fact, this obsession of mine led me to a life-threatening experience one November when, yes, I got in the bath drunk. I don't mean that I was blotto or anything, but I got home one night and thought I'd dip myself into some hot water at 44 degrees Centigrade to warm myself up.[41] I was entirely compos mentis and conscious.

But something unusual happened after the first five minutes of my soak. My head suddenly got warm, and I felt severe palpitations as if my heart was thumping throughout my whole body. Shocked, I stood up to get out of the tub, and then I felt dizzy. I drank a glass of water and slumped down in the bathroom for a while. Luckily, the symptoms subsided, but for a moment I truly thought that I was going to die. This is what is known in Japan as 'heat shock'.

---

41 Translators' note: Japanese baths are often significantly hotter than Western ones.

It's said that taking a bath after drinking is a bad idea, but I never paid any attention before because I had never had a bad experience. But the November incident really brought it home to me that this was something I should never do. It was so scary that it actually stopped me drinking for a while.

But what is the basis for the no-baths rule? And what was the cause of my severe palpitations and dizziness? I put the questions to Satoshi Umemura, director of the Yokohama Rosai Hospital, who has an in-depth knowledge about heat shock and has written a book on the subject *Kōketsuatsu ni Naranai Makenai Ikikata* [*How to Live without Losing to Hypertension*].

The principle offender is sudden blood pressure change

'Heat shock is damage to the body brought about by sudden temperature change,' explains Professor Umemura. 'Change of blood pressure is deeply involved in heat shock. In particular, taking a bath in cold weather after drinking is extremely dangerous, because your blood pressure changes dramatically.'

So the cause of heat shock is the change in blood pressure! Sure, sudden change of blood pressure sounds bad for the body . . . But, how does taking a bath when it is cold or after drinking affect your blood pressure?

According to Professor Umemura, it's all about the air temperature.

'When air temperature is low, our body constricts the blood vessels to keep the temperature up, raising the blood temperature. But when the air temperature goes up, the blood vessels dilate to release heat and lower the body temperature, and the blood pressure along with it. So our blood pressure goes down in summer and up in winter.'

Changes of blood pressure before, during and after a bath

From warm room to **cold dressing room** and **bathroom**	Blood pressure **up** ↑
Soaking in the **bathtub**, the sympathetic nervous system tightens and our bodies constrict the blood vessels	Blood pressure **up** even more ↑
While soaking in the bathtub, the body warms up	Blood pressure **down** ↓
Getting out of bathtub to go to the **cold dressing room**	Blood pressure **up** ↑
Putting clothes on and going back to a **warm room**	Blood pressure **down** gradually ↓

From cold to hot, the temperature changes your blood pressure

So how does my blood pressure change when I take a bath?

If you are going from cold to warm, to a hot bath, back to cold, your blood pressure is yo-yoing so much due to the temperature changes that it makes me dizzy just thinking about it. That's what causes the heat shock. In fact, the graph shows the measured fluctuations in blood pressure in the course of a bath. It is clear that the lower the room temperature is, the bigger the change in your blood pressure when you get into hot water.

'Sudden blood pressure change is hard on the body,' says Professor Umemura. 'Having a bath when it is cold places a heavier burden on the body because the change is so great. It's particularly bad for the elderly, as they may have high blood pressure anyway, or have developed arteriosclerosis. In other words, their blood vessels are already damaged and fragile. They have a higher risk of being unable to respond to a sudden change in blood pressure, which in turn increases the possibility of a heart attack, stroke or cerebral haemorrhage. Also, older people have less ability to keep their blood pressure stable through positional change (lying down, sitting down, standing etc.), so they have an increased risk of fainting when they stand up in the tub, because the blood doesn't get to their head fast enough.'

Changes in blood pressure during bathing

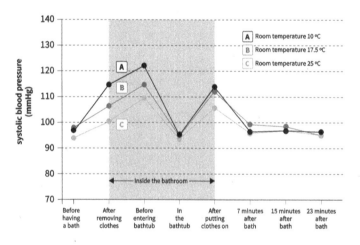

Blood pressure change is significant when having a bath, but if the room temperature is low, the swing becomes even greater. (Kanda K, Ohnaka T, Tochihara Y, et al., 'Effects of the thermal conditions of the dressing room and bathroom on physiological responses during bathing' in *Applied Human Science Journal of Physiological Anthropology*, Volume 15, 1996, 19-24).

Winter is the high season for accidental deaths in the bath

Data released by the Japanese Consumer Affairs Agency indicates that there are many accidental deaths at bath time in the cold season from December to March. Most of the victims are elderly people over sixty-five years of age. Accidental bath deaths in Japan have risen 1.7 times in the last decade.

Seasonal change in accidental death during bathtime in twenty-three Tokyo wards

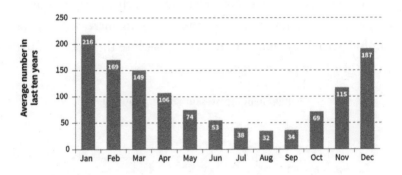

(Consumer Affairs Agency: 25 January 2017 press release)

Hmm, it looks like we should not underestimate the danger of bathing in winter. Because most of the Japanese soak in the bathtub instead of taking a quick shower, Japan has by far the highest numbers of bathtub deaths in the world.

According to Consumer Affairs Agency's 2015 research into the reality of accidental deaths at bath time in winter, about 10 per cent of the people surveyed said they had been shaken by feeling dizzy or losing consciousness during their bath time. Many of the respondents reported the symptoms occurring when they stood up in the bathtub after 'soaking in the bath water for long time (longer than 10 minutes).'

'When you soak in bath water for a long time,' explains Professor Umemura, 'your blood pressure lowers. If you try to stand up suddenly in that state, blood vessels usually try to constrict to stabilise the blood pressure, but when you are old, your body cannot stabilise the blood pressure and because the blood does not circulate into your head enough, you faint. If you happen to fall in the bathtub, you could end up drowning.'

Alcohol temporarily lowers your blood pressure

So far, I've learnt how taking a bath in winter, where there is a huge gap between the room temperature and the water temperature, is a burden for the body. But we haven't got round to the drinking part, yet, as this is without taking alcohol intake into consideration. How dangerous is it, then, to take a bath after drinking alcohol under the same conditions?

'Drinking alcohol temporarily lowers the blood pressure,' says Professor Umemura. 'Drinking alcohol increases the blood concentration of acetaldehyde, the alcohol metabolite, which dilates the blood vessels and lowers your blood pressure. We believe that when the blood pressure drops, the sympathetic nervous system (SNS) reacts to try and stabilise it by increasing your heart rate.

'If you're drinking, then your blood pressure is even lower than normal, and so getting in the bath causes an even bigger fluctuation. Combine a bath, and winter, *and* drinking and the danger mounts up. And of course, if you are drunk, you have foggy reasoning and lower ability to manage a crisis, which increases the risk even more.'

Listening to that, I can understand the causes of the heat shock I experienced. I'd lowered my blood pressure through drinking, and then I'd gone from a warm room to a cold bathroom, and jumped in a hot bath at 44 degrees. My blood pressure shot up, and then dropped again through an increased heart rate. So then I stood up, with low pressure, which is what caused my dizziness. I was lucky I didn't slip or drown.

'If you were a bit older,' agrees Professor Umemura, 'you might have fainted, fallen and drowned.'

Just thinking about it makes me shiver.

Post-drinking drop in blood pressure

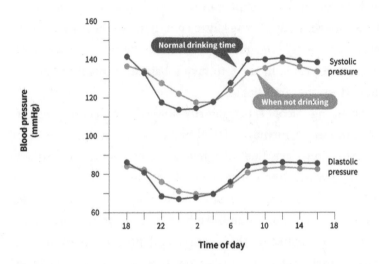

Blood pressure changes when those with high blood pressure are drinking (normal drinking time) and refraining from drinking (when not drinking). There is a tendency for blood pressure to lower when drinking at night, while the daytime pressure is up. (*Rishō Kōketsuatsu - Clinical Hypertension* - June, 2000, p.14).

Habitual drinkers have high blood pressure

Professor Umemura has worse news for those like me who drink habitually, and advises regular blood pressure checks.

'There is a strong correlation between alcohol and blood pressure,' he explains. 'The more you make a habit of drinking, the higher your blood pressure tends to be. Blood pressure increases in proportion to daily alcohol intake. This applies to everybody, regardless of their ethnic background or the types of drinks they have.'

So the aforementioned lowering of blood pressure by alcohol is only a temporary affect for occasional drinkers. If you drink day after day, your blood pressure goes up!

'Currently, there are said to be forty-three million people in Japan with high blood pressure,' says Professor Umemura. 'Blood pressure tends to go up as we age, but there is a huge number of Japanese men in their fifties who have high blood pressure through stress. Habitual drinkers may not have high blood pressure *yet*, but there is a big chance they will develop it later.'

Come to think of it, many of my drinker friends do have high blood pressure. Heavier drinkers tend to suffer from it, and it seems that many people seem to develop symptoms in their fifties. If you are one of the drinkers of the world, you can't ignore this even if your levels are currently normal.

Correlation between daily alcohol intake and blood pressure

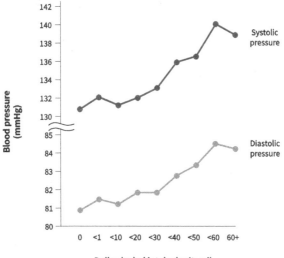

The greater the alcohol intake, the higher blood pressure becomes. Alcohol 30ml is equivalent to a 633ml bottle of beer or two glasses of wine. (M. H. Criqui, R. D. Langer, D. M. Reed, 'Dietary alcohol, calcium, and potassium. Independent and combined effects on blood pressure' in *Circulation*, Volume 80, No.3, 1989, 609-614.)

What should I do if I desperately want to have a bath?

Having learned the danger of having a bath after drinking, especially when it is cold, I am sure there are quite a few people who still want to freshen up before bedtime. Isn't there a safe way that they can?

'I realise you might want to wash,' says Professor Umemura, 'but you really should hold off getting in a bath until the alcohol has been metabolised and the after-effects have gone away. For an adult man weighing 60kg, a single unit of 20g of pure alcohol (a 500ml bottle of beer), will take about three or four hours to leave his body.

'Alcohol metabolising capacity varies from person to person, so this is only a guideline, but you should wait at least three or four hours. Those who get red-faced when drinking have lower capacity, so they'll need to wait longer. Of course, the more you drink, the longer the alcohol lingers as well, so you have to be careful.'

Professor Umemura warns that apart from leaving a gap between drinking and having a bath, we need to pay attention to the four points listed opposite. Also, having a bath soon after eating and after taking sleeping pills or tranquillisers should be avoided.

Don't use the sauna either!

Another thing to avoid after drinking is a sauna. Some people swear by 'sweating out the alcohol' in a sauna, but it's not the alcohol that you are losing, it's even more water. Even in normal circumstances, people in a sauna need to hydrate themselves. After drinking, your body is often in a state of dehydration, therefore it is extremely dangerous to dehydrate your body even more. If you drink and have bath and go to bed straight afterwards, the state of extreme dehydration will increase the risk of heart attack or stroke. People with advanced arteriosclerosis should be particularly careful.

Four things to watch out for at bath time

1	Narrow the temperature difference by warming the dressing room and the bathroom before having a bath. When running a bath, using the shower head will raise the room temperature with its steam.
2	Keep the temperature of the water below 41°C and do not soak in the water for longer than 10 minutes. Avoid a long bath. A half-body bath is easier on the heart, but the temptation to stay in for longer will eventually bring the risk up to the same level.
3	Do not suddenly stand up when getting out of the bathtub. This is an important point to prevent dizziness.
4	If you have a family member in the house, ask them to check if your bath time is longer than usual. There is a report that there are fewer cases of cardiac arrest at public baths, because other people tend to notice quickly if something goes wrong.

Professor Umemura could tell from my face that I still wanted a solution, so he suggested that the best option for reducing the risk of heat shock would be to have a shower.

'A lukewarm shower will be much easier on your body than soaking in a bathtub,' he says. 'Also, even if you faint, there is no danger of drowning. It's drowning after fainting that causes the most problems in Japan, because we have a habit of soaking in the bathtub. It's why our bathtub drowning statistics are so overwhelmingly high, compared with other countries.'

That's true! There is the alternative choice of taking shower, which is more common in other countries. I was fixated on a bath because of the mistaken idea it would 'sweat out the alcohol'. But sure, a shower seems much less risky, and even if I faint, a few bruises are better than dying. From now on, I will shower after drinking, and I will try to warm up the bathroom beforehand, to reduce the temperature difference. And I shall make sure that the water is not too hot.

A shower after drinking won't be quite the same, but it will be safer. However, I was surprised to hear that heat shock can be exacerbated by habitual drinking because of the *high* blood pressure drinkers so often develop. Of course, the real problem is *excessive* drinking, which is why we really need to stick to that old favourite, the 'moderate' amount (20g in pure alcohol conversion, or one cup of saké).

Once you hit fifty years old, you should regularly have your blood pressure checked to monitor for changes. And if you find out that your levels are on the high side, reduce your alcohol intake. At the end of the day, you are the only person who can protect yourself.

The Slippery Slope – the frightening fate of alcoholism

Expert Adviser: Yōichi Kakibuchi
Tokyo Alcoholic Medical Treatment Synthesis Center,
Narimasu Welfare Hospital

Drinkers have too many things to worry about – deteriorating liver function, weight gain, gout, memory loss, forgetting things . . . And one that surely should concern the heavy drinker is alcohol dependence, also known as alcoholism.

Many people think that you can only develop alcoholism if you drink an extraordinary amount. However, it is a surprisingly familiar and scary experience for drinkers.

I'm no exception, and I often find myself wondering: 'Am I an alcoholic . . . ?'

On my days off, I like to have a glass of sparkling wine with my lunch, and tell myself it's a little personal treat. On weekdays, when the clock strikes five, I like to crack open a beer while I am making dinner. That's totally normal for me, but when I mention it to my teetotal friends, they look at me askance and ask: *'Isn't that a slippery slope . . . ?'* It made me realise for the first time that it is not actually 'normal' to drink at lunchtime or while you are cooking.

I drink much, much less than I did in my younger days, but I still take a drink with my evening meals without a shred of self-doubt.

In spite of being old enough to know better, I still occasionally drink so much that I can't remember what happened. Am I on course to becoming an alcoholic?

I've worried more ever since I lost someone to alcoholism. He kept drinking whisky on the rocks, despite his doctor telling him he couldn't after surgery for pharyngeal cancer. But he kept knocking back the whisky, even during the day. He couldn't stop, even after his beloved wife warned him, and he passed away at fifty.

That might be an extreme example, but I am sure there are many people who worry about not being able to drink in moderation. For these kind of worries, unique to drinkers, I sought the advice of Yōichi Kakibuchi, director of Tokyo Alcoholic Medical Treatment Synthesis Center, Narimasu Welfare Hospital, about the danger of alcohol dependence and when he considers dependency to start.

1.09 million alcoholics and 9.8 million potential alcoholics!

To start with, I asked Dr Kakibuchi the current situation. How many alcoholics are there really?

'According to the Ministry of Health, Labour and Welfare research group,' he says, 'the number of alcoholics in Japan is estimated to be 1.09 million. On top of that, there's another 9.8 million "excessive drinkers", with the potential to develop alcoholism.'

I'm shocked! It's surprising to hear of over a million alcoholics, but also close to 10 million people who are excessive drinkers.[42] Dr Kakibuchi added that there are increasing numbers of female alcoholics, which made me worry even more that I might be one of them.

---

42 The Ministry of Health, Labour and Welfare research also estimated there are 10.39 million 'high risk drinkers', defined as those whose daily average consumption is more than 40g in pure alcohol conversion for men, more than 20g for women.

'Alcohol over wife!' – the terrifying truth about alcoholic dependence

But what are the 1.09 million alcoholics suffering from?

'We can't simply define alcoholism by the amount someone drinks,' says Dr Kakibuchi. 'There is no clear borderline, and it can vary depending on someone's living environment. So, rather than set a particular limit on intake, we carefully assess if drinking is causing any particular problems, such as physical illness, mental illness, violence, domestic discord, or absence from work without notice. Also, if the person is *able* to moderate their alcohol intake or stop drinking, and if the problem is persistent.'

Dr Kakibuchi leans on the World Health Organisation's diagnostics guideline from its ICD-10 (International Statistical Classification of Diseases and Related Health Problems 10th Revision). These have six items, including: a strong desire to drink alcohol; difficulties in controlling its use, such as when to start or stop drinking, or the amount; experiencing physical withdrawal symptoms at any attempt to moderate or cease drinking; and persistent drinking despite harmful consequences. If the person continuously or repeatedly experiences more than three of these situations in a year, it is diagnosed as alcohol dependence.

In reality, Dr Kakibuchi likes to establish a diagnosis by talking to the patient, their family and the people around them. He asks questions about what kind of drinking problems they are experiencing. In some cases, the problems are extremely serious and obvious, in which case there is no need to go through the diagnostics.

'Many couples come in together, but when the wife asks her husband what's more important to him, her or the alcohol, some answer "Alcohol" without even hesitating. When it reaches that level, it's the kind of alcoholism that requires immediate hospitalisation.

As you can imagine, the chances of divorce are high. In fact, it's well known that alcoholics have a high divorce rate.'

Estimated number of alcoholics and high-risk drinkers

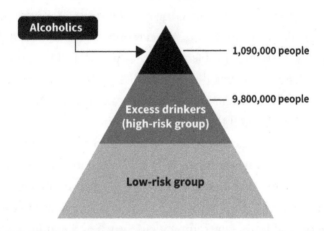

Estimate based on findings of the Japanese Ministry of Health, Labour and Welfare research group in 2013. The number of alcoholics was determined using the ICD-10 criteria. Excess drinkers are those who habitually drink over 60 grams in pure alcohol conversion.

Choosing booze over your wife . . . I don't need WHO guidelines to tell me that is alcohol dependency. There are some people who keep drinking even after a divorce and broken home, after they've been sacked by their company, without any income and living on the dole, but they just keep drinking until they die alone.

Terrifying. Before I get to that point, I shall try not to go any higher than the 'high-risk group'. Except I am already there . . .

Watch out if you drink more than three cups of saké a day

So what kind of people are categorised in the high-risk group?

'For example, they might be those who habitually consume a large amount of alcohol with high liver function value (gamma-GTP).

They get told at a health check that it's risky, and they briefly stop drinking and lower the value, but then go back to the previous drinking amount. They have had alcoholic hepatitis for years, but they manage to work and don't have any problems at home, and are not experiencing any other noticeable drinking problems.

'Such people are one step away from alcoholic dependence, but they do not need to stop drinking immediately. They do require expert help to reduce the amount that they drink.'

And with 9.8 million Japanese people in the high-risk group, it's not that small a number. According to Dr Kakibuchi, there are many businesspeople who fall within the category. As for the daily intake, he says that 60g in pure alcohol conversion is the line.

'I'm sure that many people are already aware that a moderate amount is usually thought to be about 20g in pure alcohol conversion – one cup of saké or a 500ml bottle of beer – for Japanese men. That's a low-risk level. But the more you drink, the more the risk, and if your intake goes over 60g, that's when drinking problems start to appear and people should seriously think about moderating the amount they drink. The experts call it the "60g Wall". Once you get to 80g, there will definitely be problems.'

In pure alcohol conversion 60g is three cups of saké. It is an easy amount for the drinkers. Even if you do not have any drinking or health problems now, the risk of becoming an alcoholic in the future is high. They are indeed potential alcoholics – and in Japan, it's not unusual for salarymen, the kind of businessmen out on works 'entertainment' outings, to have a liver function gamma-GTP value of over 300. According to the Japan Society of Ningen Dock, a rating over 101 is considered abnormal.

'I heard a story at a society meeting from the health management section at a major company,' says Professor Kakibuchi. 'They decided to offer health guidance to anyone at the company who had a gamma-GTP of over 300. But so many people at the company had scores over that level that there was no time to schedule all the sessions, so they revised the danger level to 500. A gamma-GTP over 200 is considered highly elevated, and over 500 as extremely highly elevated. It went to show that there were many potential alcoholics in the company, even though they appeared to be working normally.'

Apparently, among those who are hospitalised for alcoholism, the liver function can be so bad that the gamma-GTP values have risen to 4000.

The drinking habit screening test

I am sure that there are now quite a few drinkers reading this wondering if they are okay? What about me? How do I know? There is a simple test for determining if your drinking habits have put you on a slippery slope.

'Firstly,' recommends Dr Kakibuchi, 'try the World Health Organisation's AUDIT – the Alcohol Use Disorders Identification Test. There's also KAST, which stands in Japanese for the Kurihama Alcohol Dependence Screening Test, provided by the Kurihama Medical and Addiction Center. They don't diagnose you, but they can help you identify the level of your drinking problem.' There's a copy of AUDIT on page 225.

So, I tried it right away. There are ten questions altogether, asking about normal drinking habits of the past year, and the result comes in a few minutes. My mark was seven points, which was lower than expected, but . . .

'They are only guidelines, of course,' says Dr Kakibuchi. 'But if you score under nine points, you are low risk. If you score between ten and nineteen, you are at high risk (potential alcoholism). If you score over twenty, you are a suspected alcoholic.'

Visualise your alcohol intake

In order to avoid an unhappy ending, those in the high-risk group need to look after themselves. They shouldn't go any higher on the scale, and, if possible, should reduce their alcohol intake until they drop to a lower category. But what can they actually do to achieve that?

'Keep a record,' says Dr Kakibuchi, 'and try to visualise your alcohol intake. That's the key to moderating the amount that you drink. I suggest that people keep a record of five data points – (1) your target alcohol intake, (2) what you drank and how much, (3) did you achieve your target? (4) did you have two consecutive liver resting days? (5) did you do any exercise?

'The important thing, is that once you're keeping a list, make sure everybody around you knows about it. When you do that, it is difficult to prevent a more moderate drinking habit, particularly if you show it to your spouse or family members and ask them to check it for you. Also, you can write in the gamma-GTP values from your regular check-up, as well.'

Dr Kakibuchi stresses that it is also important to decide what you want to gain by meeting the target. That can be anything, from improvement in gamma-GTP values to a better marital relationship.

'In short,' he says, 'anything that you feel is worth the reward.'

Unreasonable targets can cause a rebound

So how should we decide on our alcohol intake?

Dr Kakibuchi cautions against setting an unreasonable goal, as that will only cause a backlash. In fact, it's unreasonable to expect someone guzzling 60g of alcohol a day to suddenly drop it to a moderate 20g. It is more reasonable, and achievable, to do it in steps, such as aiming for 40g, and then doing that for a few days, and then dropping to 30g.

'Just as though you were on a diet,' says Dr Kakibuchi, 'just how much you're drinking becomes clearer when you write it down. You will get support from your family. There are many people who have regained their health by keeping a record of their alcohol intake.'

In fact, one report has shown that six months of lifestyle recording can pay huge dividends. Fifty-five male drinkers, who either scored over ten on the AUDIT survey or who habitually ingested more than twenty-one drinks per week (210g of pure alcohol), were selected and given specific health guidance. Over six months of recording their drinking, they experienced noticeable reductions for AUDIT points, alcohol intake, abdominal circumference, body weight, diastolic blood pressure, ALT and gamma-GTP. Meanwhile, their good cholesterol (HDL) went up. Out of fifty-five participants, forty-nine (89.1 per cent) had metabolic syndrome at the start of the test, down to thirty-one (56.4 per cent) by the end.[43]

Dr Kakibuchi says that alcoholic dependent patients 'tend to be stubborn and not to listen to other people. Otherwise, they would have listened to the people around them and succeeded in reducing or stopping their drinking *before* they had to come to the hospital.' But if the results are as clear as these figures, wouldn't even a stubborn person decide to give it a try? Even I feel like I can keep up with this.

Is there anything else we need to be careful about in order to prevent becoming an alcoholic or potential alcoholic?

---

43 Iyadomi, M. et al. 'Tokutei hoken shidō no wakugumi o riyō shita high-risk inshu-sha ni taisuru shokuiki ni okeru shūdan sesshu shidō (S-HAPPY program) no kōka' [Effects of a Group Alcohol Intervention (S-HAPPY Program) at the Workplace for High Risk Alcohol Drinkers Using the Framework of the Specific Health Examination and Health Guidance System of the Metabolic Syndrome] in *Rōdōkagaku* [*Journal of the Science of Labour*] 2014; 89(5): 155–165.

'Drinking habits can progress,' says Dr Kakibuchi, 'from occasional drinking, when you drink at special events, to habitual drinking, when you drink even if there are no events, to compulsive drinking, when you don't care about the time or the place.

'Even if your alcohol intake stays the same and you have not experienced any particular harm from drinking, if you feel like you are missing out on something when you are *not* drinking, there is a possibility of "usual-dose dependence". That is, as it were, a medium risk. And then, when you start increasing drinking amount or time, with excuses such as "I feel lonely", "because it's my day off", or "because I cannot sleep", it becomes high-risk and it is harder to turn back.'

Hmm . . . Sounds like I have to warn myself off having a day-time drink just because it's my day off.

To keep us from a sad ending to our lives, those of us who are aware that we are drinking too much should keep a record of our alcohol intake. We should work out where we stand, and make efforts to reduce the amount we drink. If at all possible, try to get as close to the moderate amount of 20g per day in pure alcohol conversion.

But in any case, why don't you take the AUDIT test for starters, and see where you end up?

The Alcohol Use Disorders Identification Test (AUDIT)

1.	How often do you have a drink containing alcohol?
0	Never
1	Monthly or less
2	Two to four times a MONTH
3	Two to three times a WEEK
4	Four or more times a week

	2. How many drinks containing alcohol do you have on a typical day when you are drinking? (one gō of saké is equivalent to two drinks)
0	One or two
1	Three or four
2	Five or six
3	Seven, eight or nine
4	Ten or more
	3. How often do you have six or more drinks on one occasion?
0	Never
1	Less than monthly
2	Monthly
3	Weekly
4	Daily or almost daily
	4. How often during the last year have you found that you were not able to stop drinking once you had started
0	Never
1	Less than monthly
2	Monthly
3	Weekly
4	Daily or almost daily
	5. How often during the last year have you failed to do what was normally expected from you because of drinking?
0	Never
1	Less than monthly
2	Monthly
3	Weekly
4	Daily or almost daily
	6. How often during the last year have you needed a first drink in the morning to get yourself going after a heavy drinking session?
0	Never
1	Less than monthly
2	Monthly
3	Weekly
4	Daily or almost daily

	7. How often during the last year have you had a feeling of guilt or remorse after drinking?
0	Never
1	Less than monthly
2	Monthly
3	Weekly
4	Daily or almost daily
	8. How often during the last year have you been unable to remember what happened the night before because you had been drinking?
0	Never
1	Less than monthly
2	Monthly
3	Weekly
4	Daily or almost daily
	9. Have you or someone else been injured as a result of your drinking?
0	No
2	Yes, but not in the last year
4	Yes, during the last year
	10. Has a relative or friend or a doctor or another health worker been concerned about your drinking or suggested you cut down?
0	No
2	Yes, but not in the last year
4	Yes, during the last year

From the Ministry of Health, Labour and Welfare e healthnet (http://www.e-healthnet.mhlw.go.jp/information/dictionary/alcohol/ya-021.html)

Amount of alcohol: 'one gō of Sake = two drinks', 'a 633ml bottle of beer = two and a half drinks', 'one glass of double shot Whisky-and-water = two drinks', 'one glass of shōchū-and-hot-water = one drink', 'one glass of wine = one and a half drinks', '1 small glass of plum wine = one drink'.

Epilogue from Dr Shinichi Asabe – Although there are many pleasures in life . . .

This is a rich, full-bodied, flavoursome book. And it's a valuable, definitive book, with a wide range of topics including many detailed expert interviews and up-to-date information about drinking and health.

If you look on the internet, you'll find a mixture of wheat and chaff, cut-and-pasted information from ambiguous sources, along with adverts from health supplement companies. It is difficult to know what is correct and what is not.

We all need a certain level of literacy, not only for information on drinking, but on general health, which is why this seriously written book is so precious.

In Japan, the amount of drinking steadily rose in step with post-war economic growth, but it has stagnated since the 1990s. Alcohol consumption among adults has been declining ever since somewhere around the year 2000. Drinking by women is slightly on the increase, but among men, particularly in the younger generation, it has been dropping.

There are many reasons for this, including the divergence of entertainment and communications with the spread of the internet, changes in health awareness, and a reduction in the old habits of work-related drinking. Undoubtedly, a part of it has been the dissemination of more knowledge about the relationship between alcohol and health.

In this book, the author interviewed many experts, not only on the dangers of drinking, but about the possibility of health benefits, and means of minimising the impact of alcohol on the body. Reading through it as a doctor, I am prompted to reiterate that drinking does come with a risk of many illnesses. Much of this data is backed up by observational studies of large groups, and speaking scientifically, I can say that the level of corroborating evidence is high.

Conversely, when we look at claims about drinking's positive effects, most of them seem to be based on experimental cell research or studies of small groups, and the majority conclude that there is a 'possibility' of health benefits, but that it is still 'debatable'. Undeniably, the level of evidence is not as strong.

The famous 'J-Curve' phenomenon indicates that a small alcohol intake can reduce the risk of cardiovascular illness; however, as a whole, the harm from drinking should be obvious, along with the fact that a moderate amount is c.20g per day in ethanol conversion (one 500ml bottle of beer, or one cup of saké). For drink lovers like us, this is rather a strict standard. But based on current knowledge, you should keep your consumption at this 'moderate' level if you value your health.

In the meantime, the effects of drinking on the body vary quite widely from person to person. It is difficult to give a standard ruling because we have different genes, influencing the enzymes that metabolise alcohol, as well as factors such as our body size, gender and age.

Also, we live with many risks. If you are a 'zero risk taker', who wants to remove every possible danger to living a longer life, then I cannot recommend drinking for you. But most people accept certain levels of risk and enjoy their lives. The most important thing is to avoid excessive risk.

This book will give those who choose the health risk of 'drinking' a chance to enjoy it and a hint about what the acceptable risks might be.

Not everyone needs to live a zero-risk life. And 'taking a health risk' really means being actively aware of our own health. There are many ways to receive an SOS signal sent by our bodies, such as a regular check-up, and paying attention to the test results.

On top of that, much of the expert advice is hardly surprising. Have a balanced diet, watch your salt intake, hydrate, don't eat too many calories, watch your weight and exercise. Avoid the double risk of drinking and smoking, which has a synergistic effect. Enjoy a moderate amount of alcohol for you, and have some non-drinking days to avoid addiction, and to give your liver and brain a rest.

And if a test shows that your liver function value has declined, you have to reduce your alcohol intake or give up drinking altogether. This should all be a matter of course, and if you make the effort to try, even just a little at a time, to follow these guidelines, I believe that even those who love to drink can do so healthily.

It's important that we drink happily.

Shinichi Asabe, hepatology specialist
Department of Gastroenterology, Internal Medicine, Jichi
Medical University Saitama Medical Center, AbbVie GK

Expert Interviewees

Research collaborators

Masashi Matsushima

Professor of gastroenterology at the Department of Internal Medicine, Tōkai University School of Medicine. Graduated from the Faculty of Medicine, University of Tokyo in 1985. After a senior residency in gastroenterology at Shōwa General Hospital and a spell as a physician's assistant at the Former First Department of Internal Medicine, Faculty of Medicine, University of Tokyo, he became a researcher at the University of Michigan. After coming back to Japan, he worked as a lecturer and then an associate professor of gastroenterology at the Tōkai University School of Medicine. Subsequently, he became the deputy head of Tōkai University Tokyo Hospital and the head of its Gastroenterology and Liver Centre. In 2013 he became a professor of gastroenterology at the Department of Internal Medicine, Tōkai University School of Medicine. In 2014, he became the head of Tōkai University Tokyo Hospital. Since 2016 he has been based at Tōkai University Hospital.

Yukio Takizawa

Professor Emeritus at Akita University. Born in 1932 in Nagano Prefecture, he graduated from Niigata University Graduate School of Medicine in 1962. Doctor of Philosophy. In 1964, he became an assistant professor at the same school. In 1973, he became a professor at the Faculty of Medicine, Akita University. In 1995 he became Director-General at the National Institute for Minamata Disease. He is an adviser to the Institute and Professor Emeritus at Akita University. He has been researching the correlation between saké and health, and written many books, including *Two Gō a Day: How to Stay Healthy by Drinking Japanese Saké* [*Ichinichi Nigō: Nihonshu Iki-iki Kenkō-hō*].

Ryūsuke Kakigi

Professor at the National Institutes of Natural Science, National Institute for Physiological Sciences. After graduating from the Kyūshū University School of Medicine in 1978, he worked at Kyūshū University Hospital (Internal Medicine and Neurology), and Internal Medicine, Saga Medical School, Faculty of Medicine, Saga University. After studying at the University College London Medical School from 1985 to 1987, he worked at Saga Medical School, Faculty of Medicine, Saga University and since 1993, he has been a Professor at the National Institutes of Natural Science, Okazaki National Research Institutes (currently the National Institute for Physiological Sciences).

Toshiyuki Kusuyama

The head of the Tokyo Voice Clinic Shinagawa Otolaryngology. Graduated from the Keiō University School of Medicine. He subsequently worked at the Department of Otorhinolaryngology, Head and Neck Surgery, Keiō University School of Medicine, and became the deputy head of the Tokyo Voice Center, at the International University of Health and Welfare. He opened the Tokyo Voice Clinic Shinagawa Otolaryngology in 2010. He is a specialist registered with the Oto-Rhino-Laryngological Society of Japan and the Japan Broncho-esophagological Society. He is a council member of the Japan Society of Logopedics and Phoniatrics trustee member, and convenor and secretary of the Society of East Japan Phonosurgery. He is a part-time lecturer at the Kunitachi College of Music Faculty of Music.

Matsuhiko Hayashi

Professor and head of the Apheresis and Dialysis Center, Keiō University Hospital. Graduated from the Keiō University School of Medicine in 1977, and after a period as a researcher in Internal Medicine, at the Department of Medicine at the University of Chicago, he became chief physician of the outpatient clinic, Department of Internal Medicine (Nephrology, Endocrinology and Metabolism) at Keiō University Hospital in 1991. Since 2001, he has been a consultant at the same department. In 2009 he became a consultant at the Central Dialysis Room (now Apheresis and Dialysis Center) and a professor at the same university. He is a Fellow of the Japanese Society of Internal Medicine, Board-Certified Nephrologist and Educator of the Japanese Society of Nephrology, Fellow of the Japanese Society for Dialysis Therapy, Board Certified Senior Member of the Japanese Society for Dialysis Therapy, a Diplomate in Primary Care and Instructor for the Japan Primary Care Association.

Hiroyuki Hayashi

The director of the Shibuya DS Clinic, Tokyo. Doctor of Philosophy. Graduated from the Jikei University School of Medicine. After serving as the medical director for Plastic and Reconstructive Surgery, Tokyo Kōsei Nenkin Hospital, he opened the Shibuya DS Clinic, specialised in medical weight loss, in 2005. He is a diet specialist with an interest in pedagogical approaches to correct dieting without rebounds.

Shōichirō Tsugane

The director of the Center for Public Health Science, National Cancer Center. Doctor of Philosophy. After graduating from the Keiō University School of Medicine in 1981, he studied public health at the Keiō University Graduate School of Medicine. He was the chief researcher on a multi-purpose cohort study to research and investigate the correlation between Japanese lifestyle (including diet, drinking and smoking) and the onset of diseases, such as cancer, over a long period of time. His publications include *Recent Developments in Cancer Prevention Based on Scientific Evidence [Kagakuteki Konkyo ni Motozuku Saishin Gan Yobōhō]*.

Susumu Higuchi

Director of the National Hospital Organisation Kurihama Medical and Addiction Center. Graduated from the Tōhoku University School of Medicine in 1979. After working at Nagai City General Hospital in Yamagata Prefecture, he moved to Neuropsychiatry at the Keiō University School of Medicine. In 1982, he started working at the National Sanatorium Kurihama Hospital (now the National Hospital Organisation Kurihama Medical and Addiction Center), becoming the chief physician in its Department of Psychiatry in 1987. In 1988, he studied at the National Institutes of Health (NIH) in the US. In 1997, he became clinical research director and then assistant director of National Sanatorium Kurihama Hospital, before becoming director in 2012. He is the chairman of the Japanese Society of Alcohol-Related Problems. The head of WHO Collaborating Centre for Research and Training on Alcohol-Related Problems, a WHO expert commission member (for drug dependency and alcohol-related problems), and former chairman of the International Society for Biomedical Research on Alcoholism (ISBRA).

Yōichi Kakibuchi
Director of the Tokyo Alcoholic Medical Treatment Synthesis Center, Narimasu Welfare Hospital. Graduated from Faculty of Medicine, University of Tsukuba Graduate School in 1990, and obtained his PhD. After working as a resident at Tsukuba University Hospital, he started to work at the Narimasu Welfare Hospital in 2002. In addition to being a physician, he also gives lectures for the Japanese Psychiatric Nurses Association, local health centres and self-help groups. He was an editor of *Selfcare Series: How to live with Alcohol [Alcohol Kōshite Tsukiau]*. He is the chairman of the Japanese Society of Alcohol-Related Problems, and deputy head of the Network to Establish and Promote the Basic Act on Measures Against Alcohol-related Health Harm.

Hirofumi Ōkoshi
Chairman of the Travel Medicine Center Nishi Shimbashi Clinic since 2008. Graduated from the Jikei University School of Medicine in 1981. After working as a resident, he became an assistant in Internal Medicine at the Jikei University School of Medicine, a research fellow at the University of Washington, and principal doctor at Medical Services for Japan Airlines International. He is an industrial physician for Idemitsu Kōsan, Kyōdō News, and Fast Retailing, chairman of the Japanese Society of Travel and Health, a councillor for the Japan Society of Aerospace and Environmental Medicine, member of the JAXA Human Medical Research and Development Ethics Review Committee, a representative for the Japan Society for Occupational Health, auditor for the NPO

Health Tourism Organisation, and part-time lecturer at the Jikei University School of Medicine.

Naohiro Furukawa

Professor at the Faculty of Health Science and Technology, Kawasaki University of Medical Welfare. He worked as an assistant at Kawasaki Medical School from 1979, becoming a lecturer there in 1997. He was appointed to his current position in 2007. His specialities are the 'autonomic nervous system regulatory mechanism of enterokinesis and peptic juice secretion' and 'the neural mechanism of vomit induction'. Currently, he is researching the physiology of enterokinesis. He is affiliated with the Physiological Society of Japan.

Tetsuya Mizoue

The head of the Department of Epidemiology and Prevention, Center for Clinical Sciences, National Center for Global Health and Medicine. Graduated from the University of Occupational and Environmental Health School of Medicine in 1988. After serving as an assistant at the Institute of Industrial Ecological Sciences, University of Occupational and Environmental Health, and an assistant professor in preventative medicine at the Kyūshū University Graduate School of Medical Science, he became the head of department at the National Center for Global Health and Medicine (epidemiological statistic study), and in April 2017 he was appointed to his current position. His main areas include the epidemiological study of lifestyle illnesses, international school health, and industrial health.

Kyōko Shimizu

Associate professor at the Department of Internal Medicine and

Gastroenterology, Tokyo Women's Medical University. She started working at the Department of Internal Medicine and Gastroenterology, Tokyo Women's Medical University, in 1984. After studying at the University of Rochester in the US in 1991, she was appointed to her current position in 2009. She specialises in the treatment of pancreatic and biliary tract disease, acute pancreatitis, chronic pancreatitis, autoimmune pancreatitis, pancreatic cystic fibrosis and pancreatic cancer. She is a councillor for the Japan Pancreas Society, chairwoman of the Pancreas Research Foundation of Japan, and a fellow, instructor, trustee and Kantō branch councillor for the Japanese Society of Gastroenterology.

Seigo Nakamura
Professor of Breast Surgical Oncology, Shōwa University School of Medicine, the head of the Breast Center and the head of the Center for Clinical Genetics, Shōwa University Hospital.

Graduated from the Chiba University School of Medicine in 1982, he started working as a resident at the General Surgery Department St Luke's International Hospital. He worked as a resident at the MD Anderson Cancer Center in the US in 1997. In June 2005, he was appointed as the head of the Breast Center and a consultant in Breast Surgical Oncology, St Luke's International Hospital, appointed to his current position in 2010. He is the chairman of Japan Surgical Society, and the chairman of the Japanese Breast Cancer Society.

Shigeo Horie
Professor at the Department of Urologic Surgery, Juntendō University Graduate School of Medicine. Graduated from the Faculty of Medicine, University of Tokyo, in 1985. He obtained a United States medical license in Texas. After returning to Japan,

he worked at the National Cancer Center and in 2003, became the head of the Urology Department at the Teikyō University School of Medicine. Since 2012, he has been Professor at the Department of Urologic Surgery, Juntendō University Graduate School of Medicine. He is an instructor for the Japanese Urological Association. He was the chairman of the Japanese Society of Men's Health and Japanese Society of Anti-ageing Medicine. His publications include *Feel Motivated! The Ultimate Men's Health Medicine [Yaruki ga Deru! Saikyō no Dansei Igaku]* and *Depressed? It Might be the Male Menopause [Utsu ka na? to Omottara Dansei Kōnenki wo Utagainasai]*.

Kazue Yoshino

Director of the Yoshino Women's Clinic, gynaecologist, clinical psychologist. Graduated from Teikyō University School of Medicine in 1993, started working at the Department of Obstetrics and Gynaecology, Graduate School of Medicine, University of Tokyo in 1995. After working at Aiiku Hospital, Japanese Red Cross Society Nagano Hospital, and Fujieda Municipal General Hospital, she opened the Yoshino Women's Clinic in 2003. Assistant Chairman of the Women's Clinic Network, committee member on the Professional Women's coalition for Sexuality and Health. She appears on *Asaichi*, an NHK morning programme, as an expert in the menopause and female hormones.

Hiroyuki Sumi

Professor emeritus, Kurashiki University of Science and the Arts. Doctor of Philosophy. Graduated from the Tokushima University Graduate School of Medical Sciences in 1974. He worked at the Department of Chemistry, Faculty of Science, School of Science, Kyūshū University (biochemistry), as an overseas researcher at the Michael Reese Hospital and Medical Center, and then back in Japan at the Ministry of Education, Science and Culture, before becoming an assistant professor of physiology at the University of Miyazaki Graduate School of Medicine in 1982. Since 1997, he has been professor and dean at the Department of Life Science, Kurashiki University of Science and the Arts. He is the president of the Okayama Tempeh Society. He is known as a leading figure in research into the functionality of fermented food including *nattō*, and the fibrinolytic activity of the components of authentic *shōchū*.

Michikatsu Sato

Institute of Enology and viticulture, Yamanashi University Graduate School. After graduating from Faculty of Agriculture, Tōhoku University, he started working at the Mercian Corporation. Following a stint at the Faculty of Agriculture in the University of Tokyo and at the University of California, Davis, he became the director of the Mercian Corporation, Laboratory of Enology and Viticulture, Wine & Spirits Research, conducting further research into polyphenols in red wine. He has been the director of Research and Development Center, Alcohol Department, New Energy and Industrial Technology Development Organization (NEDO), a specially appointed professor at the winery worker lifelong training centre at the Institute of Enology and Viticulture, Yamanashi University Graduate School, and a visiting researcher at the Fruit Tree Research Station, Yamanashi Prefecture. He has published numerous papers about wine and polyphenols.

Saeko Wakazuki

Store operation department manager, Development Division, Fukumitsuya. After working as shop manager for an apparel brand, she moved to Fukumitsuya as shop manager for the newly opened SAKE SHOP Fukumitsuya Tamagawa branch. In 2010, she was involved in the opening of the SAKE SHOP Fukumitsuya Tokyo Midtown branch as the manager. She has been in her current position since 2014.

Yasuhisa Ano

Researcher, Kirin R&D Health Technology Laboratory. He obtained his Ph.D. at the University of Tokyo Graduate School of Agricultural and Life Science. He has been researching the health benefits of food, such as the dementia prevention effect of Camembert cheese. He won the Japanese Society of Veterinary Science Veterinary Science Young Investigator Award in 2014, and in 2016 was awarded the Cabinet Offices top prize for *ImPACT Healthcare Brain Challenge*.

Miki Satō

Director of the Shimbashi Sleep Mental Clinic. Doctor of Philosophy. After graduating from the Jikei University School of Medicine in 1997, he started working at its Department of Psychiatry. He worked with outpatients at the Department of Psychiatry, Jikei University Hospital, offering medical care in sleep disorders and everything in the psychiatric field. He specialises in hypnology, carrying out medical practice and researches in hypersomnia (narcolepsy, etc.), insomnia, sleep-wake rhythm disorders, etc. In particular, he is researching treatment methods combined with cognitive behaviour therapy for treating insomnia. In 2010, he obtained his Ph.D. for a study in insomnia treatment. In the same year, he opened the Shimbashi Sleep Mental Clinic.

Hisashi Iijima

Chief of the Chiba Pharmaceutical Association Drug Information

Center. Graduated from the Nihon University School of Pharmacy in 1994. Pharmacist. Doctor of Philosophy (pharmacy). After being a senior researcher at the Chiba Pharmaceutical Association Drug Information Center, he was appointed to his current position in 2007. He is the chairman of the Japanese Society of Drug Informatics, and an assistant chairman of the Promotion Committee for Clinical and Epidemiological Research, Japan Pharmaceutical Association. He is also a licensed practitioner in acupuncture and moxibustion, and a licensed leader of safe infectious waste disposal. He carries out scientific research to improve the coordination of local healthcare and quality of medicine, taking measures based on his research.

Tatsuo Yamamoto
Professor of Dental Sociology, Stomatology Course, Department of Oral Science, Kanagawa Dental University Graduate School of Dentistry. Graduated in Dentistry at the Okayama University Graduate School of Medicine, Dentistry and Pharmaceutical Sciences. Before his appointment to his current position, he worked as an assistant in preventive dentistry at the Okayama University Dental School, a visiting researcher at the Center for Biomedical Research, University of Texas, and a lecturer at Okayama University Hospital. His speciality is social dentistry, social epidemiology, preventive dentistry, oral hygiene, and oral health science. He is a winner of the 8th Biennial International Meeting of the International Academy of Periodontology John O Butler Travel Award, and the Japanese Society for Oral Health's Lion Award, among others.

Satoshi Umemura
Director of Yokohama Rōsai Hospital, Professor Emeritus of Yokohama City University.

Graduated from the Yokohama City University School of Medicine in 1975. After working as an assistant professor at the Midwest Hypertension Research Center, Creighton University School of Medicine, US, he became a professor at the Second Department of Internal Medicine, Yokohama City University School of Medicine in 1998, Dean of the School of Medicine in 2008, the head of Yokohama City University Hospital in 2010, and Provost of the Association of Medicinal Science, Yokohama City University. He has been in his current post since April 2016. He has published many books including *How to Live without Losing to Hypertension [Kōketsuatsu ni Naranai Makenai Ikikata]*.

Index

Note: page numbers in **bold** refer to diagrams, page numbers in *italics* refer to information contained in tables.